THE
DE-STRESS
DIET

THE DE-STRESS DIET

The Revolutionary Lifestyle Plan for a Calmer, Slimmer You

CHARLOTTE WATTS AND **ANNA MAGEE**

HAY HOUSE

Australia • Canada • Hong Kong • India
South Africa • United Kingdom • United States

First published and distributed in the United Kingdom by:
Hay House UK Ltd, 292B Kensal Rd, London W10 5BE.
Tel.: (44) 20 8962 1230; Fax: (44) 20 8962 1239.
www.hayhouse.co.uk

Published and distributed in Australia by:
Hay House Australia Pty. Ltd, 18/36 Ralph St, Alexandria NSW 2015.
Tel.: (61) 2 9669 4299; Fax: (61) 2 9669 4144.
www.hayhouse.com.au

Published and distributed in the United States of America by:
Hay House, Inc., PO Box 5100, Carlsbad, CA 92018-5100.
Tel.: (1) 760 431 7695 or (800) 654 5126; Fax: (1) 760 431 6948 or (800) 650 5115.
www.hayhouse.com

Published and distributed in the Republic of South Africa by:
Hay House SA (Pty), Ltd, PO Box 990, Witkoppen 2068.
Tel./Fax: (27) 11 467 8904. www.hayhouse.co.za

Published and distributed in India by:
Hay House Publishers India, Muskaan Complex, Plot No.3, B-2,
Vasant Kunj, New Delhi – 110 070. Tel.: (91) 11 4176 1620; Fax: (91) 11 4176 1630.
www.hayhouse.co.in

Distributed in Canada by:
Raincoast, 9050 Shaughnessy St, Vancouver, BC V6P 6E5.
Tel.: (1) 604 323 7100; Fax: (1) 604 323 2600

A catalogue record for this book is available from the British Library.

ISBN: 978-1-84850-779-1

Printed in Australia by McPherson's Printing Group

CONTENTS

ACKNOWLEDGEMENTS

We would first and foremost like to thank the many pioneering and brilliant clinicians and scientists whose ground-breaking work has been quoted in this book, and whose ideas and vision have been instrumental in shaping *The De-Stress Diet*. Without their work, our research and understanding of nutrition, the nature of stress and the relationships between stress and weight gain – and much more – would simply not have been possible. To name a few: Professor Carol Shively, Dr Mark Mattson, Dr Matthew Edlund, Dr Loren Cordain, Professor Robert Sapolsky, Dr Bart Hoebel and Professor Leo Pruimboom.

Our special thanks goes to the nurturers and supporters of our vision for how we hope *The De-Stress Diet* will transform people's bodies, minds and lives. Most notably, our thanks goes to our excellent Hay House editor, Carolyn Thorne (the picture of slim and calm in the face of stress), who saw the potential in our early – and enormous – manuscript. Her perseverance has been essential to the making of this book. We would like to thank our text editor, Barbara Vesey, for her intelligent input and sympathetic manuscript changes, as well as Robert Caskie at the PFD Agency, for encouraging us to begin a process that would ultimately take years to nail down and finally complete.

This book would not have been possible without the exceptional input of our trusted consultants. Fitness trainer Charlene Hutsebaut (charlenehutsebaut.com) brought her authority, experience and knowledge of modern movement, anatomy and fitness to Chapter 10, making it the effective package we hope it becomes for the reader. Nutritional cooking consultant Tina Deubert has brought a wealth of food preparation knowledge, passion and instinct to the recipes and cooking advice in this book. Her practical approach has been priceless.

All illustrations are by the very talented Jackie Coulson, whose lovely yoga teaching shows in her drawing style.

We would also like to thank the entire team at Hay House, including Jo Burgess, the energetic publicity director, for transferring her obvious enthusiasm and belief in the book to the media, as well as Jessica Crockett, Jo Lal, Julie Oughton, Amy Kiberd and Leigh Fergus for their invaluable contributions to its publishing.

Our writing and brainstorming sessions took place at the British Library and we must thank their canteen staff for the most fantastic fresh steamed sea bass, vegetable and chilli dishes they cooked from scratch for us (always with a smile), and the café staff downstairs for patiently putting up with our fussy post-lunch coffee orders.

Charlotte would like to thank those who have provided the most applicable and inspirational nutritional, naturopathic and functional medicine knowledge along her continuing educational journey: Marion Kirkham ND, Chris Astill-Smith, Dr Nigel Plummer, Dr Robert Verkerk, Dr Jeffrey Bland, Lyra Heller, Stephen Terass, Jules Cattell and Alessandro Ferretti of Equilibria Health, Nutri-Link Education and the Institute for Optimum Nutrition. Both on a personal and spiritual level, Jim Tarran – her yoga teacher of 15 years and founder of the Vajrasati Yoga School – and his persistence with authenticity, exploration and finding what we might need rather than want. Also, her great friends and yoga inspirations Khadine Morcom and Leonie Taylor, for their caring and having babies at the same time to provide true empathy. Charlotte would like to thank her partner, Sam, for giving her the time to fit in this book by being the great fun and caring modern dad that he is, her dad, Peter, for always turning up to save the day and provide subversive merriment, and most of all to her daughter, Maisie, for being the loveliest source of 'good stress' and providing fun, cuddles and constant hilarity.

Anna would like to thank her phenomenal inspiration Leslie Kenton, whose health books fuelled her health-writing ambitions at age 14, along with Suzanne Wangmann, Trish Halpin, Frances Power, Helena Lang, Charlotte Moore, Tessa Hilton, Victoria Young, Brian Brennan and Irene Feighan for being visionary editors and encouraging Anna to pursue and research all those health ideas and features over the last 15 years. She would also like to thank her all her yoga mentors, most notably Susannah Hoffmann for her support and intuitive teaching. Anna's husband, Kevin, put up with Anna's 'tippety-tapping' away for entire weekends and well into many long nights while this book was being written, rendering their social life non-existent. She is also grateful to her father-in-law, Eamon 'The Guru' Magee, for his guidance on all things, to her dad, Peter, and sisters, Tanya, Rea and Penny, for their endless enthusiasm. Most of all, Anna would like to thank her mum, Lina, for reading all her scribbles from age seven onwards and telling her daughter over and over what a great talent for writing she's always had (regardless of whether it's true).

INTRODUCTION

It's no secret that stress isn't healthy. This epidemic of the modern world is an underlying cause of low energy, loss of sex drive, depression, tooth-grinding, high blood pressure, skin problems, infertility and insomnia. What is perhaps more staggering is how bad we are at dealing with stress: 12.8 million working days are lost to stress every year[1] and 1.5 million people are dependent on benzodiazepines (highly addictive anti-anxiety drugs whose brand names include Ativan, Valium, Mogadon and Lubrium).[2] Although almost all of us complain about feeling stressed at work, one study found nearly a quarter take no breaks, and a third turn to comfort eating and extreme dieting to cope.[3] Now, mounting evidence has shown that one of the most insidious side effects of chronic stress is weight gain. Excess stress hormones in the body encourage fat storage, especially that hardest-to-shift type – weight around the middle. Quite simply, in a stressed body most diets are doomed to fail.

The De-Stress Diet, based on nutritional therapy used successfully with hundreds of stressed, overweight people, as well as a strong body of scientific research, resets this system in your favour. It will show you calming techniques, targeted nutrition and intelligent exercise to alleviate stress *and* help you release excess weight and keep it off. We like to call it 'Slim and Calm Living'.

The De-Stress Diet Mission

- To help you reconnect with your body and release excess weight while enjoying a better quality of life.

- To give you a complete lifestyle plan to cope with stress and lose weight long term.

- To show you how to enjoy eating and preparing fresh, whole food every day.

- To encourage you to let go of feeling that you should constantly be doing something to achieve what you want.

- To teach you to ask yourself 'How will this make me feel?' when it comes to food and movement, instead of 'How will this make me look?' The De-Stress Diet makes you feel great and, as a by-product, you can lose weight and see your mood, skin and muscle tone improve.

We have taken meticulous care to ensure that everything in this book is shown to be effective by giving you references and scientific commentary. We have also called on the added expertise of exercise specialist Charlene Hutsebaut and nutritional food consultant Tina Deubert. That's why throughout this book you'll find 'Lab Chats' (like the one right here) and 'DSD Tips' to help you.

Lab Chat: *Stress and Weight Gain*

'When we are stressed our bodies create the stress hormone cortisol which encourages the body to release calories, fat and energy into the bloodstream', says Professor Carol Shively, a lecturer at Wake Forest University School of Medicine in the US who specializes in the link between fat and stress. For the last 25 years Professor Shively has been researching the effects of simulated stressful environments on primates. Stress is not harmful when it is short term, she explains.

'But when our stress is chronic and never lets up — whether that's through nasty bosses, endless work deadlines or family pressures that just never relent — our systems become flooded with cortisol and two fat-promoting chain reactions occur. First, cortisol signals the body to store fat around the belly, something that has *been observed in both animal and human studies. Second, excess stress and cortisol also make us crave sugar and fat, which is why we tend to choose junk or 'comfort' food such as chocolate or crisps when we're under stress. Stress is the missing link in the weight-loss equation that needs to be addressed.*[4,5]

Quiz: How Stressed Are You *Right Now*?

Take this quiz to see how well you're coping with the stress in your life at this moment. You can come back to it regularly and use it as litmus test to gauge your stress levels.

Your Behaviour

Do you:

react to situations or events in a more dramatic or heightened way than you afterwards think you should have?

ALWAYS ☐   OFTEN ☐   SOMETIMES ☐   NEVER ☐

feel overwhelmed if any task or demand you didn't expect occurs suddenly?

ALWAYS ☐   OFTEN ☐   SOMETIMES ☐   NEVER ☐

feel demotivated and as though every chore is a bigger mountain than it was say, a year ago?

ALWAYS ☐   OFTEN ☐   SOMETIMES ☐   NEVER ☐

feel compelled to take on more and more, even if you don't think you can handle it?

ALWAYS ☐   OFTEN ☐   SOMETIMES ☐   NEVER ☐

feel angry, scared, anxious or irritable – or swing from one to another?

ALWAYS ☐   OFTEN ☐   SOMETIMES ☐   NEVER ☐

tend to take things on for others, regardless of your time limits and feelings?

ALWAYS ☐   OFTEN ☐   SOMETIMES ☐   NEVER ☐

feel the need to 'just keep going' or to juggle all your balls in the air?

ALWAYS ☐   OFTEN ☐   SOMETIMES ☐   NEVER ☐

avoid relaxing and letting go more and more?

ALWAYS ☐   OFTEN ☐   SOMETIMES ☐   NEVER ☐

avoid difficult situations, people or crowds – even if you know, deep down, you might enjoy them?

ALWAYS ☐   OFTEN ☐   SOMETIMES ☐   NEVER ☐

seek out exciting situations, exercise or hobbies that are high risk?

ALWAYS ☐   OFTEN ☐   SOMETIMES ☐   NEVER ☐

How You Feel

Do you:

feel sensitive to bright lights, sudden noises and/or touch?

ALWAYS ☐   OFTEN ☐   SOMETIMES ☐   NEVER ☐

feel unable to filter out different sounds in a room?

ALWAYS ☐   OFTEN ☐   SOMETIMES ☐   NEVER ☐

feel less and less able to cope?

ALWAYS ☐   OFTEN ☐   SOMETIMES ☐   NEVER ☐

want to hide from the world more and more?

ALWAYS ☐   OFTEN ☐   SOMETIMES ☐   NEVER ☐

find yourself frowning, sighing or yawning often?

ALWAYS ☐   OFTEN ☐   SOMETIMES ☐   NEVER ☐

find yourself snapping at people more and wishing you hadn't?

ALWAYS ☐   OFTEN ☐   SOMETIMES ☐   NEVER ☐

feel upset more and more easily at the slightest things?

ALWAYS ☐   OFTEN ☐   SOMETIMES ☐   NEVER ☐

feel more vulnerable, fearful about the future or lacking in confidence?

ALWAYS ☐   OFTEN ☐   SOMETIMES ☐   NEVER ☐

get less pleasure out of things you used to love?

ALWAYS ☐   OFTEN ☐   SOMETIMES ☐   NEVER ☐

find small tasks harder and harder to complete?

ALWAYS ☐   OFTEN ☐   SOMETIMES ☐   NEVER ☐

How You Cope

Do you:

use stimulants such as tea, coffee, cigarettes, alcohol, chocolate, sugar or recreational drugs as a 'fix' to keep you going or to ease the pressure?

ALWAYS ☐   OFTEN ☐   SOMETIMES ☐   NEVER ☐

crave sugar, caffeine and the 'buzz' of achievement to feel alert and fulfilled?
ALWAYS ☐   OFTEN ☐   SOMETIMES ☐   NEVER ☐

watch TV, play video games or surf the net as a way to switch off or feel numb?
ALWAYS ☐   OFTEN ☐   SOMETIMES ☐   NEVER ☐

turn to behaviour such as excessive shopping, sex, drinking binges or arguments and find yourself relishing the drama or buzz?
ALWAYS ☐   OFTEN ☐   SOMETIMES ☐   NEVER ☐

do large amounts of exercise – more than one hour a day or strenuous exercise for five or more days a week with little rest?
ALWAYS ☐   OFTEN ☐   SOMETIMES ☐   NEVER ☐

sink into phases – such as entire weekends – of couch potato slump?
ALWAYS ☐   OFTEN ☐   SOMETIMES ☐   NEVER ☐

go through cycles of bingeing and overeating alternated with going on restricted diets?
ALWAYS ☐   OFTEN ☐   SOMETIMES ☐   NEVER ☐

seem to get addicted to behaviours or substances more easily than you used to?
ALWAYS ☐   OFTEN ☐   SOMETIMES ☐   NEVER ☐

feel compulsive about certain things, for example cleaning, being organized, your iPhone or social networking habit, or have an overarching need to control the outcome of things at work?
ALWAYS ☐   OFTEN ☐   SOMETIMES ☐   NEVER ☐

have a very low or exceedingly high appetite?
ALWAYS ☐   OFTEN ☐   SOMETIMES ☐   NEVER ☐

What's Going On

Do you:

grind your teeth at night and/or clench your jaw during the day?
ALWAYS ☐   OFTEN ☐   SOMETIMES ☐   NEVER ☐

have difficulty getting to sleep, or wake with a start in the small hours?
ALWAYS ☐   OFTEN ☐   SOMETIMES ☐   NEVER ☐

find concentration, multitasking or remembering things more difficult than usual?
ALWAYS ☐   OFTEN ☐   SOMETIMES ☐   NEVER ☐

feel fuzzy, confused or disconnected?
ALWAYS ☐   OFTEN ☐   SOMETIMES ☐   NEVER ☐

feel wired or on constant alert?

ALWAYS ☐   OFTEN ☐   SOMETIMES ☐   NEVER ☐

experience sudden drops in energy or constant fatigue?

ALWAYS ☐   OFTEN ☐   SOMETIMES ☐   NEVER ☐

need to sleep more and more?

ALWAYS ☐   OFTEN ☐   SOMETIMES ☐   NEVER ☐

feel unrefreshed in the morning or have to press the snooze button over and over before getting up?

ALWAYS ☐   OFTEN ☐   SOMETIMES ☐   NEVER ☐

get sick when you go on holiday or catch every infection going?

ALWAYS ☐   OFTEN ☐   SOMETIMES ☐   NEVER ☐

find yourself holding your breath or sighing unwittingly?

ALWAYS ☐   OFTEN ☐   SOMETIMES ☐   NEVER ☐

Your Symptoms

Have you noticed:

digestive issues such as bloating, belching or constipation?

ALWAYS ☐   OFTEN ☐   SOMETIMES ☐   NEVER ☐

your skin breaking out or looking grey and dull, or the onset or flare-up of conditions such as eczema, acne or psoriasis?

ALWAYS ☐   OFTEN ☐   SOMETIMES ☐   NEVER ☐

your skin looks prematurely aged, greyish or dehydrated around the cheeks and under your eyes?

ALWAYS ☐   OFTEN ☐   SOMETIMES ☐   NEVER ☐

mood swings, feeling low or depression?

ALWAYS ☐   OFTEN ☐   SOMETIMES ☐   NEVER ☐

you're developing inflammatory conditions such as asthma, arthritis or hay fever?

ALWAYS ☐   OFTEN ☐   SOMETIMES ☐   NEVER ☐

a tendency or sudden onset of allergies or food intolerance?

ALWAYS ☐   OFTEN ☐   SOMETIMES ☐   NEVER ☐

increased headaches?

ALWAYS ☐   OFTEN ☐   SOMETIMES ☐   NEVER ☐

excessive sweating or urination?

ALWAYS ☐   OFTEN ☐   SOMETIMES ☐   NEVER ☐

reduced libido?

ALWAYS ☐   OFTEN ☐   SOMETIMES ☐   NEVER ☐

heavy periods, PMS, menopausal or erectile problems?

ALWAYS ☐   OFTEN ☐   SOMETIMES ☐   NEVER ☐

Scoring

For every 'always' you have answered, give yourself a score of 3. For every 'often', a score of 2. For every 'sometimes', a score of 1. For every 'never', a score of 0.

What Your Score Means
10–50

Congratulations! You seem to be coping well with stress. But before you resell this book on Amazon, try out some of the practices, as they are designed to get you feeling and looking healthier overall.

50–70

You're seeing early signs of excessive stress. This is a good point to do something about it and develop new habits that could help you cope in future. It's also the point where leaving stress unaddressed could lead to more physical symptoms, such as weight gain and premature ageing.

70–100

You have been under increasing pressure for some time. The passion and energy with which you have met life in the past is starting to give way to frustration, demotivation and feeling as though everything is too much. You've come to the right place. With the diet, exercise and relaxation methods explored in this book, you can have a lust for life again in no time and look and feel better for it.

100 or over

Don't, well… stress, but do take on the advice in this book. Your coping methods might have worked in the past, but over time they have depleted your energy, mood and endocrine system so that you feel overwhelmed and increasingly as though you can't cope. This book is most definitely for you.

Using This Book

As you read this book, give yourself time and space to digest the ideas. The De-Stress Diet is designed to be your own 'nutritionist in a book' and help you connect to your body's natural wisdom about what it needs to remain slim and calm.

Chapters 1–3 explain the reasoning and evidence behind the plan, while the following chapters contain specific and targeted strategies for change. If you're the type of person who wants to know what to do – without the why – turn straight to the 6-Week Plan (Chapter 4). If you need to know why to make change, read the book from start to finish to gain an insight into the compelling links between stress and excess weight; then, when you are ready, begin the 6-Week Plan.

De-Stress: The 10 Principles of Slim and Calm Living

1. Pleasure Matters

Notions of 'no pain, no gain' and 'going for the burn' have no place in the De-Stress Diet. We now know that it is the rich sense memories that come from feeling better – not extreme diets – that make people stick with healthy lifestyles. Sense memories are the clear associations between change and feeling better that our bodies remember and that give us both a reason and the motivation to continue. By bringing you a complete programme with not only physical but also emotional benefits, you will have a powerful reason to stick with it long term *and* you will see knock-on results in the way you look. Ultimately, this is about living as nature intended – with plenty of sunlight, touch, sex, laughter, movement and high-quality food – to reach our highest levels of stress-free, pleasurable health and weight success.

2. Eat Like Our Ancestors

The De-Stress Diet is based on a hunter-gatherer diet, adapted to suit our modern lives. You will be moving towards a highly natural diet low in sugar and refined carbohydrates, designed to provide your body with optimum nourishment, energy, mood and appetite control and to help lower your stress levels. The De-Stress Diet is:

- **Sustainable** It works in the context of your life without fuss. In Part 2, De-Stress Eating Every Day, we have provided you with detailed breakfast, lunch, dinner and drinks and snacks chapters that anticipate the scenarios you face every day with practical lifestyle and diet advice.

- **Realistic** Not so strict that it sets you up to fail and leaves you feeling guilty, demotivated or hating us.

- **Tasty** Shows you how to love preparing and eating healthy, real and wholesome food, not only because it's good for you but because it makes you feel good.

- **Intuitive** Hard and fast rules only create more stress and rebellion from your body. Over time and through the 6-Week De-Stress Plan you will learn to transform your lifestyle by using the suggestions, advice and ideas that work for you by *feeling, not thinking* what you need.

- **Varied** Hunter-gatherers ate different amounts on different days and at different times, depending on their energy needs and the availability of food. In the De-Stress Diet there are no prescriptive or measured meals, only advice and suggestions. Without the blood-sugar roller-coaster of a high-sugar diet and stress cravings (see below) you will begin to become more in touch with what true hunger feels like and respond to your body's energy needs by eating more on some days and less on others at the times that suit your body. We do, however, advocate a modern measure of 'no skipping meals', to ensure no blood-sugar lows in the face of constant low-level stress.

3. Leave Cravings Behind

Moving away from relying on sugar and stress for energy is transforming. People experiencing this report energy that once felt 'jangly', impulsive and cyclical becoming smoother, more rational and consistent, as well as their being able to maintain positive mood, focus and concentration for longer. Reducing or cutting out sugary, processed foods also helps you break cycles of craving and yo-yo dieting which add to your stress and weight gain. You will be reducing grains, pulses, wheat and dairy and eating more satisfying healthy fats, quality proteins and highly nutritious vegetables and fruit. Better blood-sugar balance will help keep your mood more stable, concentration focused and your appetite satisfied without sugary snacks and drinks. Part of this principle is about learning to identify the ways many unhealthy foods masquerade as 'good for you' with hidden sugars and processed fats. In time, you will be able to spot insidious sugars and junk simply by reading a label.

4. Know Yourself (and the 'Stress Suit' You're Wearing)

When stress is long term and chronic, varying symptoms develop depending on body make-up. One person might break out in hives while another becomes hyper-manic. This is the specific 'Stress Suit' he or she wears. In Chapter 2 you can do a quiz to find out which suit you're wearing at any given time. We also encourage you to try the advice and suggestions in this book for a few weeks – at least – and see what works for you by feeling and observing the way your body reacts in terms of energy, mood, sleep quality and weight. Through this increased self-awareness you will discover the fundamental lifestyle and diet principles that work for *you* – not your friend, partner or know-it-all work colleague – by feeling their effects. This is about getting in touch with how your body feels and your intuition, so you can understand what you need as an individual. That makes it much more likely you'll stick to it.

5. Increase Good Stress

Not all stress is bad; scientists have now confirmed that the right kind of stress can have a positive effect on the body. Intermittent good stress and less unhealthy, chronic psycho-social stress (or, learning to manage our reactions to unhealthy stress better) is one of the cornerstones of The De-Stress Diet. This system is not always about being comfortable, though. We'll also be encouraging you to step out of your comfort zone and actively seek out healthy stressors every day.

6. Lay the Foundation

Mornings make days in De-Stress Diet terms. By reclaiming your mornings and starting the day with a nutritious, protein-based breakfast and a few simple, calming techniques, you allow your body to find its natural rhythms so it becomes stronger and more able to cope with your stressful daily life. With this comes freedom from food-obsessing and, ultimately, fewer urges to snack along with stronger connection to your own optimal energy and appetite patterns.

7. Make Time

Finding space in our hyper-connected, over-subscribed lives – even if only for a few moments a day – to do nothing, take some conscious breaths or simply feel our feet on the ground is essential to this plan. During the De-Stress Diet you will hear a lot about mindfulness – the practice of being fully present – whether that is while you eat, during a conversation, at a work meeting, in a yoga pose or as you're washing up. It's a daily in-built meditation system that can make us feel better anywhere, anytime with little or no time commitment. The good news is that eating mindfully – with full focus on the food and taste, and no distractions from work or television – has been shown to lead to weight loss and to reduce binge eating.[6,7,8,9]

8. Move... Naturally

You don't have to exercise to exhaustion to get the body and mood benefits of exercise. De-Stress Diet exercise is about increased everyday activity. It harnesses the growing interest in hunter-gatherer fitness in sports science, encouraging you to integrate daily natural, varied movement into your everyday life. Walking, cycling, swimming and/or team sports along with regular, gentle de-stressing yoga and a short, targeted strength-training routine two to four times a week will get you feeling – and looking – great and better able to deal with the stressors in your life, without costing you your energy.

9. Rest, Not Just Sleep

One of the most important – and compulsory – aspects of the De-Stress Diet is rest. According to physiologists who study them, hunter-gatherers would have had high-activity days followed by low-activity days. This would have reduced the likelihood of crippling injuries and given the body a chance to recharge itself. Yet in the modern world we go on and on with less sleep and rest than we need. Whether it's the exercise we do or the stress we're exposed to, we are best genetically suited to a variety of activities performed intermittently and with different levels of intensity, with adequate rest in between to ensure mind and body recovery.

10. Lifestyle Default

The odd night out on the tiles or that irresistible crème brulée doesn't matter in the scheme of things when you always default to a lifestyle that supports your digestive, endocrine and nervous systems towards minimizing stress responses and balancing blood sugar. The De-Stress Diet shows you that the way you eat is part of a bigger lifestyle picture so you don't need to take an 'all or nothing' approach to your diet that only leads to more stress, unhappiness and binges. For example, if you're regularly exercising, incorporating calming breathing and yoga postures into your everyday routine and avoiding sugar and refined carbohydrates *most of the time*, going off-course now and then doesn't come with the same guilt or consequences as it might if you were constantly yo-yoing from one fad diet to the next.
Enjoy!

Charlotte and Anna

Part 1
STRESS AND YOU

Chapter 1

HOW STRESS MAKES YOU FAT AND UNHEALTHY

Pundits are fond of telling us the only path to weight loss is the simple equation of expending more calories than we take in. But the growing global obesity problem suggests that diets focusing only on calories and activity levels may work in the short term, but over time increase fat storage.[1] There is something more at work keeping 1.5 billion of the world's people over the age of 20 overweight, most of them in high- and middle-income countries.[2]

That missing link is *stress*. Too much stress over too long a period not only depletes your body of nutrients, leaving it exhausted, it also alters your body's biology, biochemistry and behaviour, making it more likely to crave and overeat sugary, junk food – and to store weight.

How Stress Affects Your Body

Sitting in a traffic jam, hearing news that your four-year-old is ill at nursery or having a boss who considers a stream of expletives an acceptable Monday morning greeting are all examples of stressful everyday situations. The term 'stress' refers to any physical, mental or emotional stimulus that provokes a reaction from the body. It can be caused by circumstances such as the nasty boss or the 10-ton workload, but it's also caused in more insidious ways by our underlying fears and worries – about losing our jobs, our homes, the people we love. The latter is something psychologists have termed 'psycho-social stress', and it's the most insidious, damaging kind.

Fight, Flight or Freeze: Your Body's Stress Response

Every time you're under any type of stress, your body will activate its immediate stress response in exactly the same way. This is a survival mechanism that evolved in humans over millions of years and there is little you can do to escape it. Whatever the crisis, person or situation, a complex cascade of hormonal, neurological and physical processes are set in motion in the brain and body (see below) – this is known as the *stress response*. Your body – intelligent piece of kit that it is – evolved to deal with this process. Trouble is, we haven't changed biologically since the days when our ancestors had sabre-toothed tigers from which to 'fight, flee or freeze'. So, each time you face a stressful situation – bad boss, marriage crisis or traffic jam – your body reacts as though it's life-threatening and kicks in its response to fight through the danger, run away from it or become crippled and do nothing. Whatever the stressor you're facing, inwardly the same things are happening in your body. But when your stressor never relents (you never slay the tiger because the tiger is your job and it's always well, *there*) the same process keeps jack-potting over and over in your body, and that is when the damage – and fat – occur.

You can't override this primal response, but you can help your reaction to become lessened and more appropriate to the level of true danger. Before we explain exactly how stress leads to weight gain, let's take a look at the ways stress affects your whole body and why its effects are implicated in so many 20th-century illnesses, from heart disease to burnout.

The Effects of Stress

Stress is not all in your head. It's a physiological reaction with physiological consequences that include chemical changes in the brain. During the stress response, the body is tense, alert and ready for action. A hormonal shot of adrenaline leads to the release of sugar stored in the liver and muscles (in a form called glycogen) for energy. This was originally designed to give you an extra burst of strength or endurance and to help you be ultra-alert and aware of your environment during an emergency. But this leads to a surge in insulin, the hormone the pancreas produces to help your body use this sugar for energy. It's likely you're not working off this energy by fleeing from sabre-toothed tigers (as our ancestors were) because in today's modern world, there isn't the same call for extreme physical responses as there was when we first evolved. You can't exactly settle a work dispute by calling Jennie from accounts for a fistfight in the stairwell, so your body is left sitting and seething at your desk while this stress response takes place. The result? Excess sugar floods through your system from stress – and from the quick-fix foods that stress can make you crave. The body then converts this sugar to fat, which it stores. If you ever get digestive issues or bloating during stressful times, it's your system prioritizing energy away from digestion and redirecting it to the muscles and brain, as it assumes you'll be responding in a physical way. Nutrients from food are absorbed less and you may crave only certain foods, or lose the desire to eat altogether, but then stuff in the entire fridge contents and give your right arm for pudding once the stressor has passed. Stress will also divert blood and energy away from sexual function, not crucial under the threat of attack and a common cause of low libido and erectile dysfunction.

When someone says 'I do well under pressure,' they are not kidding. The stress of pressing deadlines can have a physically motivating effect on the mind and body. But in the long term, constantly drawing on adrenaline-based energy causes our body's blood sugar to rollercoaster dramatically. Over time that leads to impatience, lack of concentration, weight gain and exhaustion because your adrenals – two small oval-shaped glands that sit above your kidneys – have only a finite ability to pump out the stress hormones they manufacture. Your adrenal glands need rest and renewal to function optimally and be able to release the right amounts of stress hormones when your body needs them most. Expecting them to run and run under chronic, relentless stress is like expecting your Smartphone to function without ever being recharged.

The Link Between Your Brain, Your Body and Stress

Every time you do anything, from eating a strawberry to updating your Twitter status, the brain sends messages to the rest of the body through a complex system of nerves via your spine and out to your organs and limbs. The conscious, muscular part of these actions is your *voluntary nervous system*. It governs anything you do intentionally such as put the kettle on, finish a report or run for the bus. Another side of your nervous system is responsible for the things that happen without you intending them, such as blushing or sweating. Called the *autonomic nervous system*, this is also what governs your response to stress and it has two halves: the sympathetic and the parasympathetic. When someone frightens you, a big tax bill arrives or you're working under pressure on a report due tomorrow, it's your sympathetic nervous system that releases hormones such as adrenaline and cortisol to give you the energy to handle the problem. When you're relaxed and calm, sleeping, breathing with awareness, listening to soothing music or having a relaxing time, the parasympathetic nervous system is at work rejuvenating your brain and body. So, once your stressful obstacle has passed, whether it's through getting the job done or escaping to a yoga class, it's the parasympathetic nervous system that comes in to reset the chaos from the stress response and help rebalance your system towards rest and recovery. Calming down again helps stimulate digestion, sexual arousal and blood circulation to the skin and extremities, and lowers stress hormones. It's why you look and feel better after a deeply restful sleep.

Although much of the autonomic nervous system action happens automatically, we can consciously control our breathing, our diets and lifestyle to help out our parasympathetic nervous system.

The Autonomic Nervous System	
Sympathetic Nervous System	**Parasympathetic Nervous System**
Prepares the body for 'fight or flight', emergencies and activity: release of stress hormones adrenaline and cortisol blood redirected from skin to muscles, brain and heart increased heart rate and blood pressure rapid breathing increased sugar levels in blood and muscles (to fuel 'fight or flight') increased sweating tense muscles a sudden rush of strength dilated pupils more sensitive hearing inhibition of non-essential bodily processes such as digestion, which is slowed down, and sex drive, which is lowered increased production of neurotransmitters: brain chemicals such as serotonin and dopamine that create motivation	Rebuilds the body systems and reverses the changes that the stress response induces: slows heart rate lowers blood pressure normalizes blood-sugar levels constriction of the pupils increases blood flow to the skin increases and improves digestion
What stimulates the Sympathetic Nervous System	**What stimulates the Parasympathetic Nervous System**
rage/anger fear deadline looming worry about family, job or anything at all exercise that raises heartbeat scary movies video games situations where we feel out of control e. g. flying phobias sudden shock or trauma bright lights and loud noises stimulants – caffeine, nicotine, alcohol, recreational drugs refined sugars	soothing touch meditation and meditative yoga focused breathing submersion in water massage hypnotherapy acupuncture and acupressure essential oils lying down sleep darkness foods that specifically activate it e.g. celery slow-tempo classical music (especially 60bpm music by Bach or Mozart)

You can have too much of a good thing. Too much parasympathetic activity can, ironically, damage the very systems it normally takes care of, such as digestion. Striking a neat balance between stimulation – what we call 'healthy' stress – and regular recharging rest will balance these two systems and strengthen your body's ability to manage the not-so-healthy stress in your life that you can't control.[3]

Not All Stress Is Bad

Regular doses of the stress hormones cortisol and adrenaline have a motivating effect on the body. They increase our vitality, motivation and exuberance. But their supply is finite and their effects depleting. That means each time they have been released there needs to follow a period of rest and recuperation. When we are under chronic, relentless stress, our bodies' ability to produce these vital hormones wears out. Over time, that can increase illness and depression, suppress immune function, lead to dry, prematurely aged skin, increased weight gain (especially around the middle), disrupted sleep and increased appetite. But, according to a growing school of scientific thought, taken in small doses and at regular intervals certain physical and mental stressors such as the stress that exercise places on your muscles, natural conditions like bracing cold air, and the odd pressing deadline that revs you into doing your best, may strengthen your system.[4] Building up the healthy stress in your life is a crucial element of The De-Stress Diet.

Lab Chat: *Good Stress*

'Not all types of stress are bad,' says Professor Mark Mattson, Chief of the Laboratory of Neurosciences at the National Institute on Aging in the US. 'The right kind of stress can improve length and quality of life.' Regular exposure to mild stressors, he explains, causes a defensive response in the body which leads to a building up of the body's defence systems including brain, immune, muscle and metabolism function which might otherwise decline as we age. One example of this is

the way in which weight-bearing exercise increases bone density. That strengthening process is something scientists have named hormesis, which means that by exposing ourselves intermittently to good stress, we may over time protect ourselves against further, bigger challenges by building up our body's resilience to fight back both mentally and physically. Learning to deal with the effects of stress on our bodies in balanced and positive ways is more effective than trying to eliminate the stress in our lives, which can leave us feeling inadequate and disappointed when that proves impossible. Hearteningly, a researcher named Heuther has suggested that long-term stress may cause people to reject long-held assumptions about themselves or their behaviours, and that stress can help the brain adapt to reflect the emotional and mental changes that stress might bring about. In short, some stress may strengthen us physically and also help us change the way we think and act for the better.[5,6]

Good vs Bad Stress

How can we differentiate between unhealthy, damaging stress and motivating stress that can make us stronger? Here's a guide:

Positive Stressful Challenges

- **Are within our control (or seem to be)** – that job interview might be making you sweat and shake, but there is plenty you can do about your performance such as sleep well the night before, hone your CV for the job and research the company. No, you can't control the outcome, but you can control your performance.

- **Have a beginning and end in sight** – studying for exams or producing a larger-than-life work project by a certain date are stressful, but they also have an end.

- **Are followed by a period of recuperation** – Even the most prolific entrepreneurs, athletes and pressured pros need their downtime or they risk burnout. All good stress is by definition followed by time for adequate deep rest and recovery.

Positive Stressors

- **Exercise** that challenges your body and is followed by adequate rest.

- **Stretching** that demands we learn to stay calm in the face of strong sensations.

- **Being chilly** – the science of *thermogenics* asserts that being cold helps you burn fat and is a healthy stress on our systems. Turning down the heating, cold showers, outdoor movement and specific thermogenic foods signal the body to produce 'brown fat', which encourages fat burnt as fuel, rather than 'white fat', which encourages fat storage.

- **Intellectual challenges** and problem-solving where you feel a sense of control over the situation.

Features of Negative Stress

- **Chronic and ongoing** – for example, having a bad boss, an unhappy marriage, an isolated or non-existent social life, unrewarding job or money problems that won't relent.

- **Self-judgemental** – worrying, ruminating or judging ourselves over mistakes or events.

- **Out of our control** – situations (especially jobs or relationships) in which you feel helpless have been shown as the most deeply affecting type of stress.

- **Excessive physical exertion** – without time to rest and rebuild, the stress response keeps running high and can cause continual muscle tension and prevent new muscle building.

Good Stress and Thermogenics

You will be hearing a lot about *thermogenesis* in this book. It refers to heat production by the body and relates to foods, exercise and activities that encourage the body to increase its metabolic rate by creating its own heat. All forms of *thermogenesis* represent a favourable form of stress on the body and, according to researchers such as the esteemed Leo Pruimboom, Associate Professor at the University of Gerona and Scientific Director of the Natura Foundation, thermogenics can increase our bodies' fat-burning capacity by around 10 per cent. There are three ways we can increase thermogenesis in our bodies:

1. **Exercise Associated Thermogenesis (EAT)** is the production of heat in the body during intentional exercise such as running, swimming, weight training and competitive sports.

2. **Non-exercise Activity Thermogenesis (NEAT)** is the energy expended during anything we do that isn't sleeping, eating or doing intentional exercise. NEAT includes all the involuntary ways we create heat in our bodies and thus increase our metabolic rate such as fidgeting, chatting, or typing as well as through creating intentional cold states in the body through lowering thermostats to under 22 degrees Celsius, having a quick cool shower or going without a layer of clothing on a chilly morning.

3. **Diet Induced Thermogenesis (DIT)** Certain foods also have a *thermogenic* effect on the body by encouraging heat production in our systems after we have consumed them, thus raising metabolism. Foods that have *thermogenic* effects include protein and fats as well as caffeine, chilli, cayenne pepper, citrus fruits and green tea.[7]

The Stages of Stress

In the 1930s, scientists worked out exactly what happens to the body under short- and long-term pressure when Hungarian endocrinologist Hans Selye described the body's reaction to stress as a three-stage process:

Stage One: Alarm

This is your immediate reaction to the stressor – fight, flight or freeze. When it's short term, this causes a short immune system boost, both to activate inflammation to stop us bleeding to death if wounded (remember, your body is thinking 'sabre-toothed tiger') and fight off possible infections of said wound. Today, 'fighting' might mean severe tetchiness or outbursts, and 'flight' might manifest as social withdrawal, numbing with substances such as alcohol or sugar or watching hours of TV to 'switch off'.

Stage Two: Resistance

As a stressful situation continues, physical processes happen in the body to help us adapt to the stress. Take extended pressure at work: under increased mental demands, the body, in its endless intelligence, will instinctively release more stress hormones to help us stay focused. Meanwhile the immune system is suppressed, sparing energy for the tasks at hand.

Stage Three: Chronic Stress

When stressful life events and situations continue for more than a few weeks, your body, which began by resisting the stress with gusto, begins to lose its adaptive capacity. The way this happens will be different in different people. The immune system may get stuck in inflammatory mode, leading to stress-related skin, joint and/or digestive problems, while the body's ability to fight invading bacteria or viruses becomes chronically suppressed, causing the onset of sore throats, cold sores or nasty sniffles that seem to carry on and on. (In Chapter 3 there is a quiz to help you to recognize the physical ways that stress manifests in your individual body.)

Stress is an energy-rich process, demanding an extremely high turnover of the nutrients and fuel we derive from food. But our daily energy production is finite and stress can use up our quota more quickly, as well as nutrients like B and C vitamins, magnesium and zinc we need for energy and to regulate blood-sugar levels. When blood-sugar highs and lows from stress become the norm, a common symptom is sudden waking in the wee hours. Crashes at night provoke a shot of adrenaline, waking us between 4 and 5 a.m. – not helpful when you're presenting a pitch in a few hours.

People who experience long-term stress may succumb to severe infections, increased blood pressure and heart attacks due to the chronically imbalanced immunity that prolonged stress has led to in their bodies. That's why the image of the stressed CEO who suddenly drops dead of a heart attack on the golf course is more than a cliché. Chances are he or she also had a round, thick pot-belly. Why? Because all those years of stress and pressure had another side effect: fat storage.

Lab Chat: *Piling on the Stress*

Along with looking at the physical ways stress causes excess weight, researchers are now looking at human populations and associating certain types of stress with increased weight gain. Research from Harvard Medical School surveyed over 2,500 men and women aged between 25 and 74 and found that, for men, job-related demands, financial difficulties and a low support network were most closely associated with obesity and weight gain. In women, along with job and money problems, strained relationships were associated with fat and weight gain over time.[8]

How Chronic Stress Leads to Weight Gain

If you have ever felt shame or guilt about not being able to shift weight even after dieting over and over again in the past, we hope that the following will show you how complex weight gain can be and how the stress in your life has had a very real and lasting impact on your weight.

You're probably aware that chronic stress can increase your risk of heart disease, and this is something that researchers have now proved.[9] Increased, prolonged stress and emotional, psycho-social pressure have now also been shown to lead to excess fat and obesity in not one but three ways:

1. Biological

When stress hits, the first thing the brain does is mobilize its stress response. A bit like a general preparing the troops for battle, your brain's troops are hormones and their attack route from the brain to the adrenal glands is called the HPA (hypothalamic-pituitary-adrenal) Axis. The HPA Axis is the system through which the hormones you need to deal with stress are released. This happens during your stress response when all the foot soldiers (hormones) strap on their boots and come out fighting on all fronts.

First the brain signals the adrenal glands to release adrenaline, which increases your heart rate and gets blood coursing around your muscles to give you that ready-for-anything feeling. If your brain perceives the stress continuing past the time adrenaline is 'needed' (you're still in the midst of that deadline), it needs to move to plan B. Adrenaline works for about an hour before it is broken down in the body, and if your body decides you need to stay at a heightened response your hypothalamus secretes corticotropin-releasing hormone (CRH), which then signals the pituitary gland at the base of your brain to release adrenocorticotropic hormone (ACTH) into the bloodstream. Then, ACTH tells the adrenal glands to release the major stress hormone, cortisol.[10] If stress-fighting hormones really were an army, cortisol release would signal that the troops had landed.

Cortisol, Stress and Fat

Like all our hormones, cortisol plays a part in our health. Ideally it's present at high levels in the body in the morning to get us up, and at low levels at night to allow sleep; it is a steroid hormone, made from fat, and we always have some running around our systems, governing our energy levels and metabolic rate.

Adrenaline is a protein hormone, only released in a reactive way when needed. Like adrenaline, cortisol has a purpose when you're stressed, and small amounts provide short bursts of energy, heightened acuity and increased sensitivity to stress. It's known as the hormone of focus, energy and recovery.

But while cortisol in the right rhythm is essential, too much too quickly turns nasty. Cortisol stimulates appetite[11,12] – telling the body we need to take on more fuel – and during periods of prolonged stress, an overproduction of cortisol turns those extra calories into fat. Plus, abdominal cells have more receptors for cortisol than any other part of the body, so most of that fat gets stored around the tummy.[13,14] People who produce excess cortisol tend to have bulky waistlines and apple-shaped bodies rather than pear-shaped ones. But cortisol makes you fat in other, sneakier ways, too, and even if you're not apple-shaped it could play a part in excess weight. Chronically elevated cortisol can lead to the loss of muscle tone[15] and inhibit your thyroid function,[16] which can slow the metabolism and make it more difficult to lose weight, even when you are following a healthy diet.

2. Biochemical

Anyone who has felt the power of a serious craving for crisps, chocolate or ice-cream will know there is something pretty powerful at work that can turn a grown woman or man into a sugar- or junk-seeking machine. Remember what we said about your body being a clever piece of kit? Well, this is its intelligence at work once again. Your brain under stress is in dire need of continual sugar as fuel, and of feel-good chemicals to calm it down, so it seeks out the quick, temporary fix that such foods can bring. In 2006, fascinating research from the University of Michigan revealed the link between stress and sugar cravings. Researchers presented two groups of rats with sugar pellets and put one group under extreme stress: the stressed-out rats' intensity of bursts for sugar cravings tripled.[17]

Studies of humans, too, have demonstrated that high cortisol is associated with increased appetite, and especially cravings for sugar, salt and processed fats. One study found that premenopausal women who secreted more cortisol during and after stress chose to consume more foods high in sugar and fat.[18] Cortisol influences food consumption by binding to receptors in the brain – specifically the hypothalamus, which governs the part of the HPA Axis which pumps out our stress response. This can stimulate our appetite for increased junk fats and/or sugar. Cortisol also indirectly influences appetite by regulating other chemicals during the stress response, including CRH, mentioned earlier, and a hormone called leptin which sends a 'stop eating' signal to the brain. High levels of CRH and reduced levels of leptin have been shown to stimulate appetite.[19,20]

In 2006, scientists used brain-scanning technology to prove that eating junk food is linked to the same emotional reward centres in the brain as those linked to drug addiction.[21] Take the humble Hob Nob biscuit, which, it seems, can make us feel better on a chemical level. That's because the junk fats and sugars present in it work on the stressed brain's instinctive need to calm itself down. These sugars and fats do this by releasing pain-relieving opioids (which sounds like 'opium' for a reason), calming cannabinoids (think cannabis) and serotonin (the body's natural 'happy' chemical) into the brain. Trouble is, the 'high' never lasts long and is often accompanied by a subsequent mood drop that is worse than when you started out, leaving you hungrier, crankier and possibly craving more of the same. This stress-craving cycle is a form of self-medication and, like other forms (cocaine, alcohol…), it's habit-forming. The more you do it, the more you want to do it. This habitual stress eating can lead to weight gain of the 'hard-to-shift' variety because it becomes your default way of dealing with pressure. And, unless you really do live in a cave, there's always pressure.

Stress can lead you to eating quickly and more than you'd like. This is also biochemical. The brain's chemical messengers – including endorphins and neurotransmitters such as serotonin and dopamine, as well as hormones such as noradrenaline and melatonin – influence not only how we feel and cope under stress but also help govern what, why, when and how much we eat. Under chronic stress, your body's ability to produce these essential chemicals and hormones is compromised, which makes it hard to tell when you have eaten enough. When stress instead of hunger is at the helm of your appetite, you experience blood-sugar imbalances that can turn mindless overeating into a vicious circle.[22,23]

3. Behavioural

There are two emotional systems at work in the brain when we talk about self-control: our impulses and our powers of reflection.

The impulsive self makes fast associations between a choice we face and how it will make us feel. It scans our environment for quick forms of pleasure and reward. For example, the vending machine equals chocolate equals a sugar hit equals feeling more awake and focused.

Our reflective self, on the other hand, is more concerned with planning, reasoning and long-term goals, such as making a decision to lose weight or get healthy. If you ever feel in two minds when faced with a tempting something- or someone-or-other, it could be a battle between your impulsive and reflective self. The two systems compete for control over our reaction or response to some want, be that hunger, lust, rest or whatever. Now, studies have found that when we're under stress or have been doing hours of tough mental work, our reflective self is weakened and our impulsive self is more likely to take over, making us less likely to choose what we know will make us feel better long term and more likely to choose the instantly gratifying quick fix. Even if we know full well we might not feel better about our choice tomorrow, our impulsive self renders us less likely to care.[24]

Scientists at Florida State University have now found that mental strain and stress sap the energy your reflective self requires to help you make healthier choices about your behaviour.[25] Your reflective self functions best when you're rested and relaxed. When you're stressed and exhausted, your impulsive self seizes the opportunity to take over. Say you've been working long hours preparing all week for a hugely important presentation, crunching numbers, writing and rewriting your report to get it perfect and wow your client or boss. Once the task is over, the mental strain you've been under makes it less likely you'll be able to resist quick-gratification behaviours, like the vending machine, take-away or pub. That's your impulse system at work. What strengthens your reflective system, though, is regular deep rest, relaxation and recovery, *during* stressful times as well as after they have passed. Over time, prioritizing this will strengthen your reflective self so that, when you're under pressure, it maintains its ability to help you make healthier choices.[26]

If you're stressed and overweight, it's not your fault but it is *in your power to change*. Stress makes you eat more fattening food. It makes you less able to control how much you eat and leads your body to store more fat. It also makes you less inclined to stick with the habits that nurture you and make you feel and look better. In the De-Stress Diet you will be using healthy, nutritious food, smart movement and exercise as well powerful breathing and yoga techniques to flip this system in your favour, so you have fewer cravings and produce a steady stream of feel-good chemicals naturally.

Chapter 2

WHICH STRESS SUIT ARE YOU WEARING?

The way our bodies react to stress in the short term is a primal, primitive response. But when stress is chronic and relentless, it begins to compromise our bodily functions with physical symptoms. These symptoms differ from one person to the next.[1] From catching any cold going to uncomfortable bloating or dog-tiredness, it's likely that you will notice certain clusters of symptoms in your body and mind when you're under continuous, intense stress.[2] This is the Stress Suit you wear. Maybe you've been to the doctor for a few of these signs and symptoms and been told that they're 'stress-related', but walked away not really understanding how or why. In this chapter we will link chronic, psycho-social stress with real body and mind effects, and help you address them with nutrition, relaxation, exercise and other lifestyle measures.

Stress Suits

1. Stressed and Wired

2. Stressed and Tired

3. Stressed and Cold

4. Stressed and Bloated

5. Stressed and Sore

6. Stressed and Demotivated

7. Stressed and Hormonal (women only)

The Stress Suits are not static states; many people oscillate between two or more. It is likely that you will identify with more than one Stress Suit, as our biochemistry is affected by stress across bodily systems, so decide if you want to address the most pressing concern or several at a time.

The checklists in this chapter will help you to identify the specific Stress Suit you wear at any given time. The questions are compiled using the principles of *Functional Medicine*, which looks at how imbalances in lifestyle, environment and diet can manifest in the body. This looks at you as an individual to explore underlying causes, and offer natural ways to optimize health.[3,4,5]

Take the initial 6-Week De-Stress Diet Plan and add some of the lifestyle measures listed here for whatever Stress Suit you are wearing at the time. Continue coming back to this chapter and redoing the quiz from time to time. Stress Suits can be slowly but surely progressive in severity of symptoms, so noting improvements can help assure you that your efforts are having results.

This checklist is not a substitute for a full analysis by a qualified nutritional therapist (alongside your doctor), who may also advise 'adaptogenic' supplements and tests such as an Adrenal Stress Profile, which is a saliva test to measure your cortisol and DHEA levels throughout the day. DHEA is the anti-stress hormone that opposes cortisol to help calm you down, and is associated with optimal adrenal and thyroid function. It's a good indicator of how you have been dealing with stress. Other tests for factors that can worsen stress-related symptoms can also be done, such as those detecting mineral deficiencies, heavy metal toxicity (from lead, aluminium or mercury) and stool tests. In the 6-Week Plan we recommend a multivitamin and-mineral, vitamin C, omega 3 oil and probiotic supplement to help everyone cope with the demands of modern life. Some supplementation, nutrition and lifestyle extras for your specific Stress Suit are offered here, but check with your doctor beforehand if you're on medication or if you have a diagnosed condition. All supplements should be taken with food.

Stressed and Wired

Symptoms and Signs

*   Feeling on 'constant alert'

*   Quick reactions to stressful situations

*   Little relaxation time or an inability to relax

*   Feeling the need to constantly 'do'

*   Long-term life demands and/or emotional stressors

*   Feeling more and more 'unable to cope'

*   Mood swings, irritability, thin on patience

*   Light, sound or crowd sensitivity

We all have a little bit of Stressed and Wired in us. Simply by living in the 21st century and subjecting our nervous systems to constant stimulation from sound, sights, lights, information and our 24/7 hyper-connectivity, we can be on 'constant alert' without realizing it – so this heightened, wired state can become our 'normal'.[6] But insidiously, it wears out our systems.[7] Adrenal overload, raised appetite and food cravings can lead to weight gain and lower levels of the anti-anxiety neurotransmitter gamma-aminobutyric acid (GABA), crucial for calm and clarity and often low in those with insomnia, depression and addictions.[8]

If it's not addressed with rest, recovery and nutrition, a Wired Suit can quickly turn to a Tired one (see page 23) and symptoms can take longer to recover from.

If you are a 'doer' or a 'fixer', the list above probably looks familiar. You may be used to using sheer mental strength to push through feelings of exhaustion and ignoring your body's signals of tiredness and stress symptoms. This is not a sustainable state, and having any of the symptoms above shows a need to start listening to your body and respecting the need to calm down and occasionally do nothing.[9] You may find the recommendations in Chapter 11 difficult, but this highlights how much you need to let go of the reins sometimes.

Points to Prioritize

- **Slow down – slowly** The first three weeks of the De-Stress Diet will help you relax and decrease reliance on stress, sugar and/or stimulants like coffee, alcohol and/or cigarettes for energy that could eventually push you into a Stressed and Tired Suit and closer to burnout. Learning to relax is an acquired skill that needs practice, so don't expect suddenly to be able to meditate for hours if you haven't been able to sit still for more than 2 minutes to date. A few minutes of conscious breathing in the morning or before bed can make all the difference. Use the techniques in Chapters 10 and 11 and identify the ones that work for you and that you can incorporate into your life long term.

- **Walk** This regulates the stress hormones pumping into your system without generating more (as harder exercise such as running can). Walking helps to relax tense shoulder muscles and any breath-holding patterns you might have developed from chronic stress. (See page 177.)

- **Use evenings to unwind** Look at your evening activities and routine, especially as you are making changes that may take your natural energy a while to kick in. See the advice in Chapters 4 and 8 on calming down, eating mindfully and keeping the nervous system in a relaxed state.

- **Snack on celery** Its calming effects are a traditional insomnia and anxiety remedy, making it the best snack for the Stressed and Wired type. Research into celery has shown that four stalks a day actively lower blood pressure, as the chemicals apigenin and phthalide expand blood vessels and activate the calming part of the nervous system.[10] It's a good appetite-regulator, too.

- **Avoid mercury-toxic fish** This is highly toxic, affecting the adrenal glands and thyroid to cause agitation in the nervous system, and may cause symptoms such as headaches, insomnia, anxiety and depression.[11,12] Support detoxification of mercury by adding coriander, garlic, broccoli, cabbage and watercress to your cooking.[13]

- **Replace lost stress nutrients** Zinc, iron, B vitamins, vitamin C, iodine and magnesium are commonly lost from the body during the stress response. You may be running low on these. See Chapters 4 and 8 for supplementation suggestions.

Stressed and Tired

Symptoms and Signs

- Feeling tired or unrefreshed on waking
- Increasing reliance on sugar and/or stimulants for energy
- Energy dips
- Feeling fuzzy-headed or 'daytime fog'
- Exhaustion in the evening
- Feeling cold and sluggish
- Sleep disturbances
- Fluid retention

Many people living with chronic stress tend to rotate between Wired and Tired Suits, so it's possible you'll have ticked symptoms from both in the quiz on this and page 21. For some, years of being Wired without rest and recovery can tip them over into Tired with low adrenal function,[14,15,16] followed by thyroid function upset and metabolic slowing so exhaustion results and weight loss becomes more difficult.[17]

Stressed and Tired and Stressed and Wired may seem at opposite ends of the spectrum, but most people with chronic stress show symptoms of both and may feel that they constantly lurch from one state to the other. Years of high cortisol can result in crashes that leave you unable to create energy without sugar or stimulants.[18,19] This is a sign that you need to nurture yourself and re-evaluate how you live your life.

Points to Prioritize

- **Lower the stimulants** You're probably dependent on external energy fixes like stress itself, sugar and/or stimulants like coffee, alcohol or cigarettes. It can seem difficult to give these up when they seem to be the only things keeping you going or are highly habitual, but these stimulants are part of what got you to this point and are wearing you down, using up B vitamins, magnesium, zinc and vitamin C that your body and brain rely on to create energy and deal with stress.[20] One by one, cut back as you implement the positive nutrition changes in this book. As you feel better you may want/need external quick fixes less and less.

- **Detoxify** Inefficient detoxification processes caused and worsened by stagnant metabolic waste products and toxins could be making you feel sluggish and stopping nutrients getting into your cells. See page 81 for more on detoxification.

- **Rehydrate** Dehydration can make you tired, especially if you're stressed, have poor breathing patterns and are getting little water from vegetables and fruit as well as in drinks.

- **Laugh** Make sure there is laughter and enjoyment in your life, as this naturally raises the anti-stress hormone DHEA which allows you to heal and reduces cortisol. Low levels of DHEA are associated with low thyroid function and weight gain. DHEA relies on regular movement to keep levels healthy; don't think that because you're tired you should never move. On the contrary, studies show that muscle quickly atrophies without movement and our metabolisms slow down when it seems energy production is not needed. Build up intelligently as shown in Chapter 10. Pace yourself by always resting between exercise bouts.

- **Replace nutrients** Vitamins and minerals that help to alleviate low energy include iron, B vitamins including B_{12} (see page 26), vitamin C and magnesium.[21] Plus, check if you have symptoms in the Stressed and Cold section of this chapter, as you may have compromised thyroid function and be low on iodine, too.

Energy Nutrients for Tired Suits: Iron

What

Normal supplementation range: 4–40mg daily, often found in a multivitamin and -mineral; do not take high amounts without checking levels as can exacerbate inflammation.

To treat a diagnosed deficiency 50–60mg is often recommended by doctors.[22]

Best forms to supplement: iron bisglycinate (gentle iron), glycine amino acid chelate, ferrous fumarate or gluconate are readily absorbed and cause fewer intestinal side effects.

Sources

Animal sources – haem (the form from which we can make haemoglobin in blood): red meats, fish, poultry, organ meats, eggs, dairy.

Vegetarian sources – non-haem; prunes, dried figs, sesame seeds, tofu, pine nuts, millet, beans (lentils, lima, navy, pinto, black), spinach, watercress.

Oats, soybeans and fortified cereals and breads also contain non-haem iron, but unless prepared as we suggest in the coming chapters, may inhibit absorption.

Need to Know

Low iron levels can show up as tiredness through poor oxygenation of blood and lowered production of ATP, our energy fuel.

Low mood and sugar cravings can also result as iron is needed for serotonin production[23] and thyroid function.[24]

Heavy periods may reduce levels.

Haem iron from animal food sources is much easier for the human body to absorb; high-grain diets can stop its absorption.[25] Vegetarians and especially vegans may need to get levels checked by their doctor.

Vitamin B_6 is needed for iron utilization, and vitamin C for absorption,[26] so ensure good intake of these, too.

Don't take iron in food or supplement form with calcium supplements, tea or antacids, as these inhibit its absorption.

Energy Nutrients for Tired Suits: Vitamin B$_{12}$		
What	**Sources**	**Need to Know**
<u>Normal supplementation range: 100–1,000 mcg daily</u> usually in a B-complex or multivitamin formula. Even if eating animal food sources, digestive issues can cause low levels from poor absorption; sublingual (under the tongue) or liquid forms best to supplement and often come with extra B vitamins needed. It's safe to take an extra supplement (even with other B vitamins in a B complex) during stressful times on top of levels in a multivitamin. Can be injected by GP if levels are very low. [27]	Animal (high) sources: meat, poultry, organ meats, fish, eggs, milk, dairy, seafood. Plant (low) sources of B$_{12}$ are similar but not as effective and some may even worsen B$_{12}$ deficiency: dulse, chlorella, nori, cultured and fermented bean products like tempeh, tofu, miso and also mushrooms show varying amounts. [28]	Needed for DNA synthesis, red blood cell production, serotonin production, nerve health and heart health; low levels are a form of anaemia and affect the way we metabolize fats and make energy from food. Vegetarians – especially vegans – and those over 50 can commonly be low in vitamin B$_{12}$ and suffer energy drops as a result, often showing years after low intake begins. [29] Antacid and diabetes medications can affect B$_{12}$ absorption.

Stressed and Cold
Symptoms and Signs

- Waking feeling unrefreshed
- Energy less and less
- Hearing ability dropping
- Feeling colder than others most of the time
- Fluid retention and poor circulation
- Hair thinning or loss, especially outer edge of eyebrow
- Feeling demotivated and unable to concentrate
- Hoarse voice
- Hypothyroidism (low thyroid function)

Stress affects the function of the adrenal glands as well as the thyroid and sex organs (see Stressed and Hormonal, page 39). Continual 'constant alert' and perceived danger from chronic stress tells our bodies there is a need to conserve energy for potential action. Subsequently, the adrenal glands signal the thyroid to go slow by down-regulating its output.[30] As the thyroid gland governs metabolism (the rate at which every cell in the body burns glucose and fats for fuel), lowered levels mean weight loss becomes harder and harder. When the adrenal glands are tired from years of stress, thyroid hormones can struggle to reach body tissues; constant feelings of coldness, poor circulation and fluid retention can result. Since low thyroid function has been shown to lead to heightened feelings of anxiety, this can become a vicious cycle.[31]

If you have been diagnosed with hypothyroidism, regardless of whether you have the symptoms above, taking the advice in this section along with the De-Stress Diet may help to improve how you feel. If you are on thyroxine and have had symptoms relieved by medication, supporting your thyroid naturally is still important. Have your thyroid function regularly tested with your GP to check your medication levels are still right after making changes to your diet and lifestyle.

However, many people may have had a doctor's thyroid function test that says 'normal'. That's because it's possible to have a thyroid functioning slightly short of the medical classification of hypothyroidism, or because your body is not utilizing the hormones it does make.[32] If this sounds like you, especially if you recognize three or more of the symptoms above, chances are you will benefit from the lifestyle changes recommended here that will support your thyroid.

Points to Prioritize

- **Exercise** This stimulates thyroid hormone secretion and enables your body to pick it up for use. See Chapter 10.

- **Balance blood sugar** Low thyroid function can go hand in hand with insulin resistance and weight piling on, so if you take no other advice from the De-Stress Diet, lower your sugar and refined carbohydrate intake and eat quality protein and good fats at each meal to help keep your blood sugar stable.

- **Cut back on alcohol or coffee** Cut back on or give these up for a while and see if your symptoms improve. Alcohol and coffee interfere with thyroid function and provide a hefty dose of sugar, further upsetting blood-sugar balance.[33]

- **Targeted yoga** Yoga poses like backbends or inversions (where your head is below your heart, such as Down-face Dog or Viparita Karani, see Chapter 11), encourage blood flow and delivery of oxygen and nutrients to the thyroid, while encouraging the calming parasympathetic nervous system that supports it.

- **Add amino acids** The amino acid (protein building-block) tyrosine is needed to make the thyroid hormone thyroxine with the mineral iodine (see table, below) and relies on food sources from protein and leafy greens such as curly kale, collards and spinach. Tyrosine is also used to make adrenaline and noradrenaline (these are released in immediate response to stress), which means that less is available for the thyroid.

- **Avoid raw 'goitregenic' foods** These include cabbage, Brussels sprouts, broccoli, cauliflower, turnips, mustard greens, collards and kale, which interfere with thyroid function and can cause enlargement of the gland when eaten raw.[34] However, they're extremely beneficial to the thyroid when cooked, as they support liver function – and thyroid hormones are activated in the liver.[35] Soy is also goitregenic.

- **Hot up** One of the words you will hear throughout this book is *thermogenesis,* which simply means 'heat-creating'. Low thyroid function reduces the amount of heat produced as energy in cells; thermogenesis can help this. Thermogenic activities include lowering the thermostat at home or walking outside in brisk weather so your body is forced to make its own heat. Thermogenic foods play a similar part in heating up the body and include chilis. For more see page 60.

- **Thyroid-supporting nutrients** These include iron, zinc, copper and selenium,[36,37] which may have been depleted through a non-organic, grain-rich or long-term vegetarian diet, and should be included in the multivitamin and -mineral supplement outlined in the 6-Week Plan, along with recommended food changes. Iodine is crucial for thyroid function, too.

Thyroid-supporting Iodine		
What	**Sources**	**Need to Know**
Normal supplementation range: 20–150mcg include in your multivitamin and mineral – see 6-Week Plan or Best form to supplement: kelp – this is a natural source of potassium iodide.[38,39,40]	High amounts found in mackerel, cod, shellfish, lobster. Some seaweeds such as kelp or kombu are rich forms of iodine (nori, dulse and arame usually test low). Buy organic as they have an easy affinity for toxic metals. Moderate amounts found in butter, eggs, goat's cheese and yoghurt. Note: even in iodized salt, the iodine can quickly evaporate; the good quality sea salt we recommend is not iodized.	Traditionally obtained from fish, seafood and seaweeds. Lower levels now eaten as less is used in dairy farming and bread-making processes.[41] Vegetarians and vegans may see low levels.[42] While mass iodine deficiency has been documented and linked to low growth and mental function in children, it can aggravate hypothyroidism in too high amounts, so don't just plough in willy-nilly above the amounts we suggest.[43] Discuss with your GP and increase iodine food intake with the amount in a good multivitamin, or have extra kelp as a natural source.

Stressed and Bloated

Symptoms and Signs

- Bloating and/or gas after eating
- Digestive or irritable bowel syndrome (IBS)-type symptoms worse when stressed
- Food sensitivities

- Constipation and/or diarrhoea – lack of daily 'full and satisfying evacuation'

- Headaches

- Poor digestion of fats and/or greasy or pale-coloured stools

- Frequent or long-term steroid medications, anti-inflammatories and/or antibiotics

- Previous diet high in sugar, refined carbohydrates and/or grains

Few people are aware of the impact gut health has on all other body systems, from immunity to our ability to deal with stress.[44] The inflammation, poor detoxification and hormone imbalance that can result from an unhealthy digestive environment is a stressful state for our bodies and minds.[45] That environment relies on the presence of around 7lb of beneficial or 'probiotic' bacteria (that's more than the weight of all of your skin cells). These good bacteria are quickly altered by stress, sugar, alcohol, antibiotics and steroid medications.[46,47] Lowered levels are linked to food intolerances, digestive issues such as IBS and weight gain.

During stress, not having enough beneficial bacteria in your gut may show as inflammation in those susceptible;[48] a growing body of evidence suggests a digestive link between inadequate levels and conditions such as asthma, eczema and arthritis.

The stress response immediately diverts energy, oxygen and nutrients away from the gut and skin towards the brain and muscle. This is activated by the vagus nerve, which runs direct from brain to gut, ordering an immediate muscular contraction of digestive muscles. So while digestion initially slows when stress hits, ongoing and chronic stress can cause spasm or constriction of gut muscles or uncomfortable cycles of diarrhoea and constipation as the gut struggles to find its balance. As serotonin (a mood-regulating neurotransmitter) is produced on the gut wall, digestive issues are linked with low mood and can worsen sugar cravings, which only contribute further to the problem.[49]

Points to Prioritize

- **Prioritize** *how* **you eat** More mindful, calm eating is a De-Stress cornerstone. Thoroughly chewed food has the best chance of complete digestion and less chance of causing food intolerances. It also helps the brain register 'full' signals before you have over-eaten.[50]

- **Assist digestion** Consider taking 1–2 digestive enzyme capsules with each meal over the first 6 weeks of your De-Stress Diet (and beyond, if necessary) to break down food eaten as you enhance your body's digestion by reducing stress hormones. Take in the first few mouthfuls of a meal. See de-stressyourlife.com on where these capsules can be bought.

- **Reduce stimulants** Refined sugars, stress, alcohol and excess caffeine compromise probiotic bacteria levels, which can lead to gas production, poor immunity and yeast overgrowths such as *Candida albicans*. Always wait an hour after eating heavy protein before having fruit, or gut fermentation can develop, causing gas. Stick to berries for least reaction.

- **Increase prebiotics** These are foods that feed your probiotic gut bacteria and have shown to help your gut cope with stress[51] and weight loss through appetite control.[52] You'll get loads from increasing your vegetable intake, but the highest levels of the prebiotic inulin are found in Jerusalem artichokes, chicory, bananas, garlic, onions, leeks and dandelion leaves (for weeding gardeners out there). Prebiotics have also been shown to help reduce the negative effects of a diet previously too low in omega 3 oils – which may have affected gut-healing abilities.

- **Herbs and spices** Ginger, mint, turmeric and other herb leaves and spices contain volatile oils that give them their pungent smells and have a calmative effect on the gut. Add herbs liberally to salads, and make fresh herb and spice teas rather than sugary soft drinks to lower your sugar intake. Parsley aids fluid retention and bloating as it helps rid the body of excess water, uric acid, salt and toxins by virtue of the plant chemicals it contains called *apiol* and *myristicin*.

- **Watch your gluten intake** Found mostly in wheat, but also in spelt, kamut, rye and barley and used in many processed foods and additives (such as dextrin and malt), gluten can cause gut problems. Bran has been shown to worsen IBS.[53] A severe intolerance can lead to coeliac disease, where the gut lining is damaged, but gluten has also been linked to IBS and inflammatory conditions including skin problems.[54,55,56]

- **Reduce lectin intake** Lectins are sugar-binding proteins (like gluten, above) found in whole grains, beans, dairy and potatoes as well as nightshade vegetables and peanuts. They are often involved in food allergies and sensitivities and can contribute to low energy and weight gain by disabling cells in the gastrointestinal tract, keeping them from repairing and rebuilding.[57] Some people tolerate lectins while others may find that lectins put a strain on their digestion, particularly if they are experiencing gas and bloating. In the 6-Week Plan you will be replacing lectin-rich foods with more vegetables and exploring how that makes you feel.

- **Get tested** Dairy, eggs, fish and grains are common foods that cause food intolerance, which is a delayed immune response, different to an immediate, obvious allergy. Food intolerances can change, especially as stress lowers and the gut heals. But you might want to consider an IgG blood test (which tests for the antibody that is present in food intolerance) if symptoms persist as you make changes, as they are almost impossible to self-diagnose. See de-stressyourlife.com for more details.

- **Extra measures** Ensure you take the probiotics and liver support recommended in the 6-Week Plan and, as you may also have some of the symptoms of the Stressed and Sore Suit, incorporate some of these measures into your lifestyle plan where you can.

Stressed and Sore

Symptoms and Signs

- Inflammatory conditions such as hay fever, asthma, eczema, arthritis or psoriasis

- Frequent infections including ear, nose and throat

- Irritable bowel syndrome and other digestive conditions

- Bloating, fluid retention and sudden weight fluctuations

- Frequent or long-term use of steroid medications, anti-inflammatories and/or antibiotics

- Diet high in sugar, refined carbohydrates and/or grains

- Degenerative conditions such as osteoporosis, heart disease, joint problems

- Auto-immune conditions such as MS, diabetes, lupus

There is rising awareness that low-level inflammation is at the root of many aspects of poor health, weight gain and chronic disease.[58,59] Even if you don't see obvious external inflammation, stress and poor dietary habits can set off an inflammatory cascade in tissues and blood vessels, and be part of the root cause of the symptoms listed here.[60,61,62,63]

Low numbers of beneficial bacteria in the gut, caused partly by stress, creates habitually over-reactive signalling from the gut to the immune system, resulting in inflammation and food sensitivities and intolerances. This is from low levels of the antibody secretory-IgA, one of the few anti-inflammatory mechanisms that the body has.[64] A nutritional therapist can use a stool test to see if you have low levels in your gut. Also follow the steps for gut health listed in the Stressed and Bloated section.

If you're wearing a Stressed and Sore Suit, your energy may be sapped by your immune system being on overdrive. This can cause a syndrome called 'cytokine sickness' in which the constant signalling of the body's immune messengers in response to inflammation can lead to a feeling of being generally unwell, in the form of low-level flu symptoms, low mood and skin conditions that won't shift.[65,66,67,68]

Excess fat may also contribute to inflammation, at the same time suppressing appetite-satisfaction hormones such as ghrelin and leptin and making weight loss difficult.[69] This is mostly true of hard barrel-belly fat, a heart disease and diabetes risk in the chronically stressed and apple-shaped.[70,71]

Eating quickly, not fully chewing food and/or eating when you're stressed can mean food enters the gut only partially broken down and then sits around contributing to an imbalance of bacteria, gas-production, bloating, constipation, food sensitivities and IBS. This is a recipe for toxicity and inflammation.

Points to Prioritize

- **Reduce sugar** This will reduce the production of inflammatory AGEs (advanced glycation end-products), created in response to sugar and stress and which can contribute to the ageing of every cell in the body (including the skin) by 'cross-linking' or lost movement within cells.[72] Sugar also disrupts white blood cell production, reducing your ability to fight infection.

- **Antioxidants** Our ancestors and those on traditional diets (e.g. original Mediterranean) ate high levels of antioxidants.[73] These are naturally occurring chemicals that counteract the harmful 'oxidizing' effects of stress, pollution, sunlight, eating burned (as on a barbecue) and fried foods and everyday chemicals. We need more antioxidants when exercising, too, as they become crucial for recovery and preventing the inflammation that can lead to injury. The De-Stress Diet is chock-full of foods that provide antioxidant nutrients such as vitamin C, vitamin E, beta-carotene, glutathione, selenium and zinc, as well as specific bioflavonoids and polyphenols in spices, tea, green tea and garlic along with smatterings of antioxidant-rich treats such as red wine and dark chocolate.

- **Hydrate** Dehydration can signal the production of inflammation-signalling histamine, so see the measures on pages 151–52 to prevent this contributing factor.

- **Watch lectin intake** (see Stressed and Bloated). Those susceptible to inflammation can react to the specific lectins in grains, beans and the nightshade vegetable family (which includes tomatoes, potatoes, red peppers and aubergines).[74,75] These lectins are lessened when cooked but try avoiding or reducing these foods if you have signs of inflammation, especially joint pain[76] (see Chapters 3, 4 and 6 for more information).

- **Get your omega 3 oils** Low omega 3 and high omega 6 in the modern diet can lead to inflammation. Those with conditions such as eczema, asthma, dermatitis, hay fever, migraines and arthritis may have difficulty converting plant sources of omega 3 and omega 6 into the anti-inflammatory, healing prostaglandins needed to get their full benefits. Stress and low levels of B vitamins and zinc worsen this tendency.[77,78] See page 67 for more information.

- **Try an antioxidant/anti-inflammatory nutrient complex** Look for any of the antioxidant substances in the following table. Those marked with an asterisk* are known to support good blood-sugar balance too.

Ingredients of a Good Anti-inflammatory/ Antioxidant Supplement		
Cinnamon*	Resveratrol	Co-enzyme Q10*
Bromelain	Quercetin	Alpha lipoic acid*
Turmeric/active agent curcumin*	Green tea extract/catechins*	Berry extracts/ anthocyanins*
Citrus bioflavonoids	Flavonoids like hespiridin and rutin	Glutathione*
Carotenoids; beta carotene, lutein, astaxanthin, lycopene	Green 'superfoods' e. g. chlorella, spirulina, chlorophyll	Herbs like Boswellia and Cat's Claw

Stressed and Demotivated

Symptoms and Signs

- Poor motivation and 'get-up-and-go'
- Tendency to depression
- Feeling less positive than before
- Using sugar and refined carbs for comfort
- Late-night binges or overeating sessions
- Sleeping issues
- Wanting to withdraw from the world
- Seasonal Affective Disorder

Our brains are energy-rich, demanding up to 70 per cent of our fuel intake. Stress increases this need and can also lead to cravings for quick fixes as our minds try and self-medicate to compensate for an inconsistent fuel supply.[79] This leads to blood-sugar imbalance, more cravings, mood swings and a vicious cycle of 'using' sugar and stimulants to keep our minds going. Stress, along with these craving cycles, also depletes the nutrients available to the brain such as magnesium, zinc, iron, B vitamins and vitamin C, required to create neurotransmitters such as serotonin and dopamine – or 'happy chemicals' – needed for focus, alertness and mood stability.

Those who tend towards low levels of these natural happy chemicals often get more of a kick from stimulating or numbing substances such as alcohol, junk food, recreational drugs and addictive medications such as benzodiazepines (the highly addictive Valium family). These habits, alongside stress, give us a sudden rise of the feel-good brain chemicals GABA, dopamine and serotonin, but they cause crashes later, leading to cycles of dependence and an increasing reliance on them to 'feel normal'.[80] These craving cycles also cause weight gain[81] which can lower self-esteem and feed into habits of bingeing and/or overeating.[82]

We can't say this enough: this is your biochemistry at work.[83] It's inaccurate to blame yourself or your lack of willpower. Excess weight has shown to contribute to depression,[84] so positive steps to slim and stay calm can help on many levels. Low or imbalanced neurotransmitters upset appetite regulation, intuitive eating and feelings of fullness or satisfaction – and stress exacerbates these cycles.[85] The De-Stress Diet will help you balance these naturally and lower your cravings so you feel better naturally.

Points to Prioritize

- **Protein with each meal** Ensuring consistent energy to the brain is the cornerstone of good mental health and motivation. Ensuring you eat protein with each meal ensures that the neurotransmitters get what they need to create and maintain a healthy mood, feelings of motivation and a desire to socialize.

- **Address your sugar intake** Sugar addiction cycles can be aggressive in those who tend to have low serotonin levels. Serotonin is crucial to our sleep and mood cycles, so inadequate levels trigger a survival mechanism in the form of sugar craving for a quick fix. The De-Stress Diet promotes blood-sugar balance to break this cycle.

- **Mind your gut** Explore the advice for the Stressed and Bloated Suit. Even if you don't have those symptoms, there is a strong gut–brain connection. Wheat and dairy, for example, may break down serotonin stored on the gut wall. Evidence shows that replenishing probiotic gut bacteria also helps alleviate mild depression, as the inflammation process that starts in the gut produces the immune messengers which can have depressive effects on the brain.[86]

- **Try magnesium** This mineral regulates brain and muscle functioning. Low levels are linked to depression, anxiety and lack of motivation. See page 127 for food sources and supplementation.

- **Omega 3s** DHA, an omega 3 fatty acid found in fish oil, is the most abundant fat in the brain and is known to be essential for serotonin receptors and dopamine levels. Low levels of dopamine and serotonin are linked to depression and other mental health issues.[87] See page 67 for supplementation information.

- **Get out and get moving** Sunlight and movement are two key components of robust mental health. Ironically, those who feel low and like hiding away from the world may worsen the situation by lowering crucial serotonin and vitamin D levels. Serotonin can be used to make up for a lack of the sleep neurotransmitter melatonin if we don't get enough sunlight, as melatonin is made in the body from exposure to natural daylight. This will further deplete serotonin levels.

- **Find natural highs** Natural opioids or 'beta-endorphins' are produced in response to laughing, music, socializing and sex, a fabulous reward system for keeping the species going. Unfortunately sugar causes a surge of these, too, so can be even more difficult to give up when we are not creating our own.

Vitamin D		
What	**Sources**	**Need to Know**
Normal supplementation range: 2,000–10,000IU a day is safe, 2,000 common in high-strength supplements.	Best source: sunlight. Half an hour a day in non-direct sunlight or 10 minutes a day in direct sunlight, without sunscreen, is sufficient.	Needed for mental health, bone density through calcium utilization and prevention of some cancers.[89,90,91]
Best form to supplement: cod liver oil or vitamin D_3.	High amounts found in mackerel, salmon, trout, herring.	Deficiencies arise when not enough sunlight exposure on bare skin, with high rates where heavy-factor sun creams are used.[92]
Vegetarian form: vitamin D_2 is synthetic and works less effectively than D_3, so prioritize sunlight exposure.[88]	Moderate amounts in eggs. *Note*: Cow's milk and other dairy foods are fortified in the US but not the UK.	Dark-skinned people in cold climates may need more sun exposure to produce same amount of vitamin D as light-skinned people.

Stressed and Hormonal – for Women Only

Symptoms and Signs

- PMS or a history of menstrual problems
- Periods becoming heavier, more painful, less regular
- Female hormone issues e. g. fibroids, endometriosis, PCOS
- Premenstrual or ovulation sugar cravings
- Hormonal phases of irritability, crying and/or negative thoughts
- Menopausal symptoms
- Fertility issues
- Long-term use of oral, IUD or injected hormonal contraception

If your sex hormones are unbalanced, chances are you also scored highly for some of the preceding Stress Suits. That's because your adrenal glands and thyroid directly affect the balance of oestrogen and progesterone in your body, and when they become unbalanced through stress, heavy, painful periods and other hormonal symptoms may result.[93,94] This is because cortisol and other stress hormones depend on progesterone for their production, and this can skew the delicate balance your hormonal system needs to function well and also lead to weight gain in 'female areas' like the bum, hips and thighs. Stress can also raise male 'androgenic' hormones in women, leading to male-shaped weight around the middle, menstrual and menopausal problems and polycystic ovarian syndrome (PCOS).

The De-Stress Diet optimizes your liver function, digestion and blood-sugar balance, which consequently helps hormonal regulation.[95] But we do advise that you visit a nutritional therapist for targeted personal advice and possible further testing.

Points to Prioritize

- **Liver support** Liver detoxification will increase your ability to break down and release used hormones from the body. See more on detoxification on page 59 in the 6-Week Plan.

- **Support your digestion** This also supports liver health, encouraging elimination of toxins and excess hormones via the bowel. Looking after your digestion will also help address any constipation which could be causing used hormones and toxins to be reabsorbed into the body. Try the Bircher Muesli Medley on page 90 and add in the soaked linseeds for hormone-balancing lignans.[96]

- **Eat some soy (but don't overdo it)** You might be confused about conflicting health messages regarding soy as help or hindrance for female hormone issues and menopausal health. Traditional fermented forms of soy such as soy sauce, tamari (gluten-free soy sauce), miso, tempeh and natto have long been associated with female health.[97] But traditionally, the Chinese and Japanese only ate soy once they had learned to ferment it – to reduce the phytic acid and lectins – and tofu and miso are traditionally eaten in small amounts as an accompaniment to meals containing meat or fish. Soy can particularly interfere with zinc absorption which can affect our ability to balance all hormones – sexual, adrenal, thyroid and blood-sugar balance – as well as affecting tissue-healing and fertility.[98] Practically speaking, eating small amounts of these soy foods several times weekly can help female hormone-balance regulation, but avoid soy in other processed forms like soy milk, soy protein isolate and textured vegetable protein (TVP). These are used to make 'fake' meat products, tend to be high in toxins, are usually genetically modified and can upset hormone-balancing abilities.

- **Watch the alcohol** It can raise circulating oestrogen and may worsen PMS and breast cancer risk, especially if you take it in drip-feed amounts and find that nightly glass often turns into half a bottle.[99]

- **Choose organic meat, eggs and dairy** It's more expensive but worth it, and if you can only make one organic choice make it this. Non-organic meat, eggs and dairy are higher in the growth hormones which disrupt hormone balance.[100,101]

Chapter 3

SLIM AND CALM ON A PLATE: DE-STRESS DIET OVERVIEW

For many of us, confused appetites, tastes and cravings add up to a stressful relationship with food, the very thing that should be nourishing us and allowing us to cope well with stress.

Hunter-Gatherers and Us

The De-Stress Diet is derived from a hunter-gatherer diet. According to its pioneers, such as Dr Loren Cordain, we are 'Stone Agers living in a Space Age'. Although our bodies have adapted in some ways to our modern lives and environments over the last 12,000 years (since the Stone Age), our basic physiology is still set to eat, move and live in the same way that our ancestors did.[1] The field of genetics is now understanding that our diet and lifestyle choices have an actual impact on the way our genes express throughout our lives, making us more susceptible to weight gain and disease.[2] By choosing to eat, live, move and relax in a way that is more in keeping with our ancestors' lifestyle, we can build a better resistance to modern life and the stress that comes with it.[3] This is the cornerstone of the De-Stress Diet.

Our bodies evolved to want food to provide motivation for the huge amount of time and energy our ancestors needed to hunt or gather it. Our physiology and biochemistry were established at a time when food was scarce and certainly not as easy to obtain as it is for us

41

today. Our hunter-gatherer ancestors living in the Stone Age or Paleolithic Era (pre-10,000 BC) would have worked extremely hard for each and every calorie they ate, and everything would have been unprocessed and naturally nutrient-dense. The amount of food they took in would have varied widely day-to-day, depending on food sources and energy expenditure, the latter of which was estimated to be 3–5 times that of the average 21st-century Westerner.[4] Our bodies are designed for this eat-more-some-days-less-others state, and responds well to variety in the amount and nutrients we eat. That's why sticking with the same amount and type of food for weeks or months may mean that weight plateaus and weight loss can become difficult, especially with stress in the equation.[5]

Our ancestors' diet would have been packed with levels of vitamins, minerals, antioxidants, soluble fibre and omega 3 oils that we struggle to attain with our 21st-century diets.[6,7] We know this because nutritional scientists are now looking beyond the effects of what we are eating today to learn from anthropology, archaeology and geography, as well as epidemiological studies from hunter-gatherer tribes living close to a Stone Age existence today, to work out exactly how our ancestors lived, ate and moved. This research has shown that our ancestors and those now following hunter-gatherer or Paleo diets and lifestyles have lowered levels of obesity, heart disease, cholesterol, depression, cancer, osteoporosis and inflammatory conditions such as acne. Their body composition and fitness were/are also superior, with less body fat.[8,9,10,11,12]

The advent of farming a mere 10,000 years ago changed our diet and lifestyle, introducing grains, beans, potatoes, dairy and domesticated meats and, eventually, refined sugars, fats and processed foods which rose rapidly after the Industrial Revolution from the mid-19th century onwards. But in evolutionary terms, 10,000 years is not long at all. This is the key reason our bodies are not thriving on our modern diet or living habits; true genetic adaptation takes millions of years. Some scientists now believe the Western 'diseases of civilization' have their roots in inflammatory processes and poor blood-sugar control that come as a result of our modern diet[13] which exacerbates, rather than strengthens, our reactions to the perpetual stress we're under.

Why Our Modern Diets Don't Suit Our Stressful Lives[14]

- **Low-quality fats** from highly domesticated and processed meats, dairy, refined vegetable oils and processed foods provide more saturated fats and fewer anti-inflammatory omega 3 oils than wild meat, game, fish, nuts and eggs.[15]

- **Lower protein levels** from these unhealthy fat sources promote poor body composition and a higher fat-to-muscle ratio, exacerbated by constant stress which also leads to weight gain and decreased muscle.

- **Too many carbohydrates** from grains, beans, potatoes and refined sugars and too few from vegetables, fruit and nuts can lead to more inflammation and the heightened insulin response which adds to the fat storage caused by raised stress hormones.[16]

- **Too few nutrients** from poor quality and imbalanced macronutrients (carbohydrates, fats and proteins) lead to lower levels of vitamins, minerals, antioxidants and omega 3 oils, which are also used up in higher amounts during stress.

- **Highly acidic diet** Higher sodium-to-potassium mineral levels in modern foods from fewer vegetables and fruit lead to acidity in the body. This is made worse by poor breathing patterns which happen involuntarily when we're stressed. Acidity in the body can contribute to cravings, mood swings, weight gain and bloating.

- **High-sugar, low-soluble fibre** carbohydrates such as grains and processed foods instead of vegetables, fruit and nuts heighten the blood-sugar imbalances, energy and mood 'highs and lows' caused by stress hormones.

The Modern Hunter-Gatherer Vegetarian

Where does this leave the vegetarian or vegan who may be concerned about where all this talk of 'man as predator' is going? We assure you there will be no preaching to include foods you do not want to eat – that would be a sure source of stress. Vegetarians and vegans, pay extra attention to diet and lifestyle measures as well as the supplement suggestions in each chapter to fully feel the De-Stress effects.

De-Stress Diet Liberation

We have created the De-Stress Diet to help you achieve hunter-gatherer happiness within the realities of the modern world. That's why we've married key hunter-gatherer/Paleo-type diet guidelines with other measures which traditional cultures have used, such as grains and bean meals and therapeutic foods, so you can find what suits your body best.

The De-Stress Diet

Basic Guidelines

(Also see the De-Stress Progress Charts on pages 223–31)

Adequate protein – meat, fish, eggs, nuts, some whole-fat dairy and some fully cooked legumes for satisfaction, appetite and insulin control, thermogenesis to produce brown fat instead of white 'storage' fat, immunity, gut-healing, thyroid and adrenal function

Moderate 'good' fats – meat, fish, eggs, nuts, some whole-fat dairy such as yoghurt and goat's cheese, coconut oil, avocado, olive oil, olives and butter for metabolism, energy, providing fat-soluble nutrients like vitamins A and E, heat-production to stop sugar cravings that raise insulin and signal white storage fat production, immunity, gut-healing, steroid hormone and vitamin D production

Plenty of the right complex carbohydrates – plenty of vegetables throughout the day, coconut, two portions fruit daily maximum, nuts and seeds, low grains and beans for energy production that doesn't result in blood glucose highs and lows and the overproduction of insulin and fat storage, and better mineral quantities and absorption.

Variety in the content and amount you eat on different days according to your natural appetite, energy and heat needs.

Never skipping meals – tells your body it is safe and not in a famine, although you can vary amounts and times to suit changing needs and hunger levels.

Avoiding snacking – moving away from snacking between meals as your appetite and insulin levels are regulated to give your pancreas a break from constantly working to produce insulin and digestive enzymes. For people who feel the need to snack, see Chapter 9 on healthy De-Stress snacks and drinks.

The Building Blocks: Macro- and Micronutrients

The main bulk of our food comes from macronutrients, those we need in larger amounts:

- Protein
- Carbohydrates
- Fats

We can create energy from all three, but fats and proteins are also used for the continual growth of skin, bone, muscles, organs and all body cells.

Most people think carbohydrates come only from grains, beans and potatoes, but all plant foods – vegetables, fruit, nuts, seeds – provide carbohydrates, with lactose in dairy the only animal sugar source.

Anthropological studies have noted that our larger brains and shorter digestive tracts distinguish us from other primates. Our ancestral diet is higher in brain-building proteins and fats; the level of plant foods eaten by chimps and gorillas can lead, in humans, to gas, bloating and inflammation. Fats do contain more calories than carbohydrates, however, and this has been the thinking behind the high-carbohydrate/ low-fat diets of the 1980s and 1990s.[17,18] Our lean ancestors didn't eat this way, though, and numerous studies have now linked this high-carbohydrate diet with weight gain.[19] Fat – unlike carbs – increases the satisfaction we feel long after a meal.[20]

The diet industry has fixated on ratios of fats-to-proteins-to-carbs for decades, but there is a growing realization that the *micro-nutrients* you eat – the vitamins, minerals, omega oils, amino acids and others needed in only small amounts – have a significant effect on your metabolism, mood, appetite and weight. Metabolism and weight management is not as simple as calories burned equals energy expended.[21] Our bodies' hormone levels and energy-burning rates are always changing, along with our appetite needs. Healthy adrenal glands, thyroid, brain, pancreas and liver are essential to the way your body adapts to daily demands, with stress both tiring them and depleting the amount of micronutrients they can draw upon. Nor are these micronutrients easily acquired from a high-carbohydrate, low-fat diet.

The De-Stress Diet is designed to replenish the macronutrients and micronutrients that stress uses up. However, even the healthiest of modern food is subject to poorer quality soil, more intense farming and travelling further distances than our ancestors' food did, which adds up to a less nutritionally potent package. Add stress and pollution to the equation and you can see why we also suggest certain targeted supplements.

Protein for Satisfaction and Thermogenesis

The nutritional CV of quality protein is impressive. This muscle-building, energy-giving macronutrient aids loss of stored fat, satisfies appetite and creates fat-burning heat or *thermogenesis* while promoting muscle-building.[22,23,24] Our ancestors would have eaten more and better quality sources than we do, obtaining protein from both dense, wild animal sources including meat, fish, organ meats, shellfish and eggs and from many more alkalizing plant sources. Scientists have studied tribes of people on contemporary versions of hunter-gatherer diets and found they have not only improved long-term weight loss but also lowered risk of cardiovascular disease and type 2 diabetes.[25,26,27,28] Yet current recommendations of 15 per cent calorie intake from protein are at odds with our ancestors' intake of an estimated 19–35 per cent. In the De-Stress Diet, protein is recommended at each meal. Our ancestors would have not been sedentary, and protein at every meal is important to keep sedentary muscle from atrophying, as well as keeping blood-sugar balanced and appetite sated until the next meal.

Protein and Fat Help Us Handle Carbs

The slower release of carbohydrates in a meal by the presence of slower-digesting fat and protein means better blood-sugar balance.[29] When you're under stress, this is essential. The more carbohydrates in a meal, the more insulin is needed to get the sugar – as glucose – from the broken-down carbohydrates into your bloodstream and then your cells for energy. As insulin rises, blood-glucose levels drop. A high-carbohydrate meal can result in an insulin surge, which means this drop happens suddenly. This sudden low blood glucose or *reactive hypoglycaemia* signals a need to find more food. Survival mechanisms then override rational thought, forcing the most direct route to a quick blood-glucose rise: sugar or stimulants like caffeine, alcohol or cigarettes.[30,31] This keeps us locked in the stress response described in Chapter 1, and needing to eat between meals.

Too Much Insulin, Too Much Fat

Too many sudden glucose surges into the bloodstream have a direct link to weight gain. While we can use some of this glucose as energy, and store some as glycogen in the muscles and liver, any excess beyond that is converted to fat. High insulin keeps us in fat-storing mode, and if we also move too little we have a recipe for long-term weight gain. Simply put, moderating your insulin response by eating little sugar and fewer refined carbohydrates means your body will use up stored fat more efficiently.

The highs and lows of a high-sugar and refined carbohydrate and/ or grain diet means your body and brain receive inconsistent glucose energy supplies. This can quickly affect mood and feed into sugar-addiction cycles that cause cravings, stress and weight gain. Long term, this raised insulin production can eventually lead to saturated insulin receptor sites which can no longer pick up the insulin hormone, a state called 'Insulin Resistance' or 'Metabolic Syndrome'. This is on the rise and is linked to diabetes, weight gain around the waist and heart health problems. As insulin fails to move sugars out of the bloodstream they must be converted to fat, so the likelihood of weight gain increases.[32] This is exacerbated by stress hormones but alleviated by exercise and by reducing your intake of high-insulin-response foods such as grains, dairy and sugars.[33] Many of the micronutrients in vegetables, fruits, lean meat, nuts and spices have properties that help insulin sensitivity and are an important part of the De-Stress Diet, especially if we want the occasional sugary treat.

Clarity on Carbohydrates

Our hunter-gatherer ancestors probably ate about 65 per cent plant foods. These carbohydrate sources would have consisted of vegetables, fruits, nuts, seeds and edible raw roots, which we advise you to increase as your main carbohydrate sources. Grains, cereals, beans, peas, corn and roots that need to be cooked (potatoes, tapioca, sweet potatoes, parsnips, yams) are not believed to have been introduced into the human diet in any significant quantities until farming, harvesting and cooking became common. What's more, the more obvious refined sugars and processed foods and desserts weren't a common feature until the Middle Ages. Reducing refined sugars, grains and beans and increasing vegetables as a long-term dietary change is simple and sustainable.[34]

Vegetables, Leaves, Stalks and Edible Roots

There are many properties in vegetables that help enhance the digestibility and absorption of nutrients in grains and cereals. But most people eat too many grains and too few vegetables, which can lead to digestion problems and nutrient deficiencies. For weight loss, eating many more vegetables with smaller amounts of grains and beans (or none at all) reduces the amount of insulin produced and makes the carbohydrates in the plant sources less likely to lead to fat storage.[35] Plus, the soluble fibre in vegetables, nuts and fruits has been recently associated with a loss of belly fat.[36] Our De-Stress guidelines in the chapters to come have suggestions and advice on preparing vegetables to make them more varied, tasty and interesting.

Grains/Cereals and Beans/Legumes

Grains (wheat, rye, rice, oats etc.) and beans (soy, pinto, chickpea, green peas, lentils, green beans, peanuts etc.) are relatively new to the human diet, only eaten in very sparse amounts before our ancestors stopped their nomadic hunter-gatherer lifestyles to stay in one place and culti-vate them. We have processed them more and more to move towards the modern Western diet, to a point where they dominate our diets, especially in the form of fast food.

The Trouble with Grains and Beans

Lectins

These chemicals cause the immune system to respond with inflam-mation in people susceptible, and can contribute to weight gain and digestion problems.[37] Lectins have been widely associated with *leptin* resistance – leptin is a hormone that acts as a signal to the brain to in-hibit food intake and register fullness. Lectins have been shown to bind to leptin, resulting in loss of appetite control, obesity and diabetes.[38]

Phytic Acid

This is a substance which studies have shown inhibits the body's ab-sorption of minerals such as calcium, iron, zinc and magnesium, and its ability to digest protein fully.[39,40,41] When grains and beans comprise more than 50 per cent of our diet, mineral deficiencies can result as rickets, tooth decay and osteoporosis.[42,43,44] This can be worse for those with lower levels of beneficial, probiotic gut bacteria.[45]

While refined grains such as white rice, pasta and bread are lower in phytic acid and lectins, they create an insulin surge and offer little nutritional value, so undoubtedly add to weight and health issues. If you choose to eat grains for energy purposes, switch from refined ones to small amounts of whole grains.[46]

Traditional farming cultures always neutralized these anti-nutrients by soaking, sprouting, fermenting or naturally leavening beans and grains.[47,48] This meant that any breads, porridges, stews, grain or bean flours were also cooked slowly or with natural acidifiers (see Chapter 6 for how). We'll explore what level is right for you in the 6-Week Plan, but even simply moving your vegetable-to-grain/bean ratio more in favour of vegetables has positive implications for increased detoxification, more favourable alkalinity in your blood, healthier mineral levels and more soluble fibre for a healthier gut.[49]

Moving Away from Low-fat

The weight-loss wars of the last few decades have focused on high-carb/low-fat vs high-protein/low-fat.[50] But the often recommended low-fat diet – high in vegetables, fruit and whole grains – has resulted in only a small reduction in the risk of heart disease.[51] Recommendations for the blanket reduction of all saturated fat was born of poorly reported evidence that it leads to heart disease and weight gain, when those who restrict it are shown to weigh more.[52,53,54] This focus on calorie reduction has driven general weight-loss and health guidelines to recommend that we get 30 per cent or less of our calorie intake from fats. But our hunter-gatherer ancestors derived between 28 and 58 per cent of their energy from fats.[55,56]

Not all fats are created equal. We are made of fats, especially our fat-rich brains, and they need to be replenished. But high fat intake from sources such as sedentary, grain-fed animals, and damaged 'trans' fats from fried and processed foods, pose risks of increased cancer, liver and heart disease, especially if the diet is also high in sugar.[57] This combination has shown a rise in liver disease in developed countries even in children.[58] The right fats, on the other hand, are essential to mood, weight stabilization, appetite satisfaction and overall health.

Fat Facts

Fats are energy-rich and for our ancestors would have represented more pay-off for energy spent finding them; their dense, micronutri-ent-rich sources would have kept 'stoking the fire' in terms of heat production and metabolism. Our ancestors would have eaten leaner meats from wild animals with quality muscle and naturally lower fat levels with much higher omega 3 fatty acid levels.[59,60]

Omega 3 oils contain the essential fatty acids DHA and EPA which are crucial to brain and heart health as well as mood stabil-ity. Plant sources contain alpha-linoleic acid (ALA) which needs to go through a series of conversions to become DHA and EPA, often pro-hibited by stress and nutrient deficiencies. DHA is in high levels in the brain, central nervous system and eyes; EPA supports heart and circulatory functions. Together they have important anti-inflammatory actions in all body cells. Low levels may contribute to weight gain[61] and poor fitness as they help to prevent insulin resistance, prevent degen-erative muscle loss, help regulate fats[62] and cholesterol in the liver and bloodstream, help serotonin levels to break craving cycles and help weight loss by improving satiety after meals.[63]

Omega 6 oils are high in the modern diet (from foods like cere-als, seed oils and bread) and have been shown to raise levels of en-docannabinoids in the brain. Endocannabinoids increase appetite and dampen memory, mood, pain perception and energy (yep, the same system affected by cannabis and yes, these effects similarly bring on 'the munchies' and are linked to weight gain). Eight weeks' supplementation with krill oil (rich in both omega 3 oils and also phospholipids, which nourish brain chemistry) have shown to reverse these metabolic dys-functions.[64]

Our hunter-gatherer ancestors probably received around 10 per cent of their total calories from saturated fat.[65] A recent meta-analysis does not support the risk of saturated fats for heart disease, with one study of 53,664 people showing a higher risk of heart attack when saturated fat was replaced by refined carbohydrates.[66] We need satu-rated fat in our diets to build new cells, to protect organs and for nervous system communication. When levels are low the body will produce its own from carbohydrates, which can lead to sugar cravings.

Not all saturated fats behave the same. Plant versions like MCTs (medium chain triglycerides) in coconut cannot be stored as fat in humans and so act thermogenically, raising fat-burning and metabolism.[67] These are the antibacterial and anti-inflammatory fats like lauric acid and caprylic acid,[68,69,70,71] also found in human breast milk, pumpkin seeds and butter. High dietary coconut is associated with low obesity and heart disease in cultures that eat it as part of their traditional diet, showing abilities to regulate insulin, prevent metabolic syndrome, reduce heart disease risk factors[72,73] and as a healthy addition to a weight-loss diet.[74]

The replacement of saturated fat with refined vegetable and seed oils has led to an overabundance of omega 6 oils in the modern diet, linked to inflammation and heart disease.[75] Removing saturated fat from our diets often means restricting protein sources and stable fats and replacing them with refined carbohydrates, more polyunsaturated fats (and in refined forms such as trans or hydrogenated fats) and processed foods. Without them we miss a level of appetite satisfaction that can send us towards sugar addiction.

Animal meats, dairy and eggs contain a substance called Conjugated Linoleic Acid (CLA), an anti-cancer[76] fatty acid that has also been shown to have positive effects on body composition, with reduction in total body fat and an increase in lean body mass when part of a healthy diet.[77,78] Foods from grass-fed animals are higher in both CLA and omega 3 oils than those fed hay or grain.[79] Studies have linked supplementation with lowered levels of the omega 3 fatty acid DHA, so it is better to get your CLA through grass-fed animal sources than from a supplement.

Dairy Foods and the De-Stress Diet

Dairy is another food which humans have only been eating since we began farming and domesticating animals, but it has become entrenched in our diets through years of recommended intake. We are not genetically designed to drink milk beyond early childhood, especially not that of another animal. Past the weaning age, most of us naturally lose the ability to digest lactase, the enzyme that breaks down lactose (the type of sugar in milk). It is believed that up to 75 per cent of the world's population is lactose intolerant to some degree,[80] with others probably adapted to produce lactase into adulthood because they are descended from cultures whose earliest ancestors drank milk.[81,82] Lactose has been shown to provoke a high insulin response, and the growth hormones used in mass-farmed dairy products have been implicated in chronic disease, acne and some cancers.[83,84]

As with fats, though, not all dairy is created equal. Some forms, such as goat's milk products, are easier for the gut to digest.[85] In the next chapter we give practical guidelines on how to make healthier choices in your dairy food selections.

How You Eat

In De-Stress Diet terms, *how* we eat is as important as what we eat at helping digestion and the manufacture of the essential brain chemicals and hormones we need to remain slim and calm. Here is a final word about what to take with you on your journey.

Mindful Eating

During your 6-Week Plan, you'll be encouraged to snack less and eat three meals a day. As you eat, ensure you chew every bite slowly, tasting it and savouring it. Mindfulness as you eat will also help your digestion and reduce stress-related issues such as bloating.

Don't Skip Meals

This doesn't work in the long term as the blood-sugar dips it creates kick the stress response into action and can lead to afternoon and evening binges (especially if it's breakfast you're skipping).[86] Studies have shown that human hunger defaults to three meals a day[87] and that hunger will peak at 7–8 a.m., most at noon and then again

7–8 p.m. even with no knowledge of time.[88] Regular meals help bring other body rhythms into line, particularly important for jet-lag recovery, coping with shift work and Seasonal Affective Disorder.[89] However you can vary amounts and times, listening to your body – not cravings – about how much it needs and when.

Connect to True Hunger

Research from Canada's McMaster University found that 97 per cent of women have felt food cravings as a result of something other than true hunger, and some stress eaters may have lost touch altogether with the feelings of hunger.[90] During this time, you will reconnect with real hunger and distinguish it from the false hunger of stress and blood-sugar imbalance. Real hunger comes on slowly, rarely less than three to five hours after eating, and is usually accompanied by a hollow feeling in the tummy. It's often satisfied by any palatable food. Mindless eating, on the other hand, is usually done quickly, often as a result of overwhelming feelings, and can often manifest as a craving for a specific food. That impulsive, 'Ooh, I fancy that' reaction to the sight or smell of tasty food is often false hunger. During this time, we encourage you to allow yourself to become hungry before you eat. Hunger is the stomach's signal that it's ready to eat, digest food and nourish the body. High sugar and junk fats can de-sensitize us to natural hunger and food intuition by creating unnatural and addictive body and brain responses.[91] Step back and check if you snack based on hunger or habit. If you really feel that the energy demands of your working day necessitate some nuts around 4 p.m., even with protein at breakfast and lunch, then that's the right thing for you. Use the Progress Charts (pages 223–31) and breathing exercises (pages 195–98) to explore how best to snack the least for any given day.

Part 2
DE-STRESS EATING EVERY DAY

Chapter 4

6 WEEKS TO DE-STRESS SUCCESS

Now it's time to get started on your De-Stress Diet journey, designed to kickstart a lifetime of Slim and Calm Living. For the next 6 weeks you will be taking steps to move away from a reliance on the foods and substances keeping you in cycles of craving and blood-sugar imbalance, leading to weight storage, stress symptoms and exhaustion that keep you coming back for more comfort food. On your journey, take special note of the lifestyle 'How Tos' in this and coming chapters, as good sleep and regular movement are as important as diet for your energy, mood, weight and appetite.

To help you get back in touch with your natural hunger, relationship and rhythm with food, we have divided the De-Stress 6-Week Plan into 3-week phases, with more help at de-stressyourlife.com:

- **Phase 1: Transition** During this time you will move away from the habits that are keeping you in addictive and fat-storing cycles and reconnect to your natural hunger signals. You will develop changing tastes and move away from craving sugar, salt and junk fats towards a calmer, healthier relationship with food.

- **Phase 2: True Change** You will begin to feel more connected and trusting of your instincts and will probably notice your appetite and sense of hunger are more regular and guided by your energy levels instead of your stress. Increased sensitivity to how certain foods and drinks make you feel will help you explore what suits *you*. During this time you will develop practical tools to use long term and to come back to in stressful times when you may stray towards less healthy choices.

Nutritional Guidelines

These are the basic guidelines for the 6-week De-Stress Diet Plan. Use the De-Stress Progress Charts beginning on page 223 as a daily reminder of what you need to do and as motivational tools.

Protein with Every Meal

Animal protein in the form of eggs, meat, fish and shellfish make the foundation of the kind of meal our ancestors would have eaten, to which you can add twice as many vegetables, both as salads and cooked.

- The starchy carbohydrate or grain part can be avoided or varied to individual needs (see page 76), with a daily portion of well-cooked beans the best choice.

- For vegetarians, nuts, seeds, live wholemilk yoghurt and goat's cheese can be added to salads and to the end of stir-fries or roast vegetables for quick meals.

- Vegans: see pages 110–11 to prepare grains and beans safely for higher intake.

Healthy Fats

Omega oils or polyunsaturated fats should make up the main part of your fat intake, especially omega 3 oils from oily fish such as sardines, mackerel, wild salmon and trout as well as eggs and meat from grass (not grain) fed free-range animals.

- Monounsaturated Fatty Acids or MUFAs from avocados, almonds, olives and olive oil, nuts, seeds should be included wherever you can.

- Vegans should include coconut, peanuts, Brazil nuts, cashews, pumpkin seeds and pine nuts for vital saturated fats.

- Unrefined, cold-pressed oils such as olive, flax and sesame oil can be used for dressings, coconut oil, olive oil or butter for cooking.

Plenty of Vegetables

Raw salad vegetables provide fibre and key nutrients. Have them with cold-pressed extra-virgin olive oil to absorb fat-soluble nutrients like vitamins A, E and beta-carotene.[1]

- Have as many cooked vegetables as raw. These are easier to digest.

- Dark green leafy vegetables and bitter salad leaves like spinach, watercress and radicchio should be eaten liberally to facilitate digestion.

- Have cruciferous vegetables at least four times a week. These include broccoli, cabbage, kale, pak choi, mustard leaves and Brussels sprouts. Avoid these raw as they interfere with thyroid function.

- Roots such as carrots, radishes and grated beetroot can be eaten raw for some starch energy.

- Garlic and onions should be eaten in abundance.

- Seaweeds can be added to soups and salads for iodine and other minerals (see page 29).

- Eat as many bright colours as possible for antioxidant variety.

- Don't rely on the nightshade family of vegetables as these are high in inflammatory lectins (see page 49). Eat tomatoes, peppers, potatoes and aubergines sparingly, cooking them to reduce the lectin content.

Alkalizing Foods

Vegetables, fruit, seeds, herbs and spices are all alkaline foods and can help keep us in the slightly alkaline blood pH levels at which our body works best. This helps balance acidity from stress, grains, beans and animal produce. Almonds, coconut, sesame seeds, chestnuts and pine nuts are alkaline (other nuts are acidic so balance out with more vegetables). Adding lemon juice to water and dressings can help increase alkalinity.

Liver-supporting Foods

Eat sulphur-rich foods such as eggs, watercress, garlic, onions, leeks and fennel for liver detoxification.

Cruciferous vegetables such as broccoli, cabbage, kale, cauliflower, Brussels sprouts, mustard greens, pak choi contain sulforaphane chemicals that enable you to produce antioxidant enzymes in the liver that work over and over again long after eating and are anti-inflammatory[2,3] (remember, these need to be cooked or they interfere with thyroid function).

Turmeric, green tea, avocados, raspberries and oily fish all help liver function.

Thermogenic Foods

These include proteins and fats, as well as chili, ginger, green tea, turmeric, cider vinegar, horseradish, wasabi, caffeine and chocolate (use these last two wisely – see Chapter 9). They help to heat the body and increase the metabolism alongside exercise and lower temperatures.[4,5]

Bitter Foods

Use endive, radicchio, chicory, romaine or cos lettuce and watercress in salads. Their bitter taste stimulates digestive juices when it hits the tongue.

Have bitter foods such as olives, grapefruit or bitter leaves before your main meal – these are classic starters for this reason. Lemon juice in hot water first thing wakes up digestion and appetite, and between meals keeps us alkalized.

Fresh Fruit

Eaten whole: 2–3 pieces a day.

In the De-Stress Diet we encourage you to drink little or no fruit juice (diluted if you do). Instead, eat fruit raw and whole wherever you can, sticking to only two (maximum three) pieces daily. Although it's rich in nutrients and great eaten in moderation, fruit is also high in sugars and can keep a sweet tooth alive – see best choices on page 73. If you are eating protein at a meal, try and wait at least an hour before having fruit, especially if you are Stressed and Bloated to ensure it doesn't ferment in the stomach.

Adequate Liquid

Have non-sugary, non-caffeinated drinks in between meals, as thirst dictates; choices include fresh, pure water, herbal or green tea and plenty of vegetables and fruit – see pages 151–52.

Weight Loss

You may lose more weight in the first week than any other as you shed fluid through the first stage of detoxification; our bodies also quickly adapt to change, so you may see different stages of results. This is a good reason not to weigh yourself but to rely on how your clothes fit as a benchmark. If you must weigh yourself, weekly is a good rule – but in terms of weight loss that you can maintain, 1–2lb a week is the healthiest speed for dropping the excess. A stone (14lb) a month maximum is a healthy goal.

As you increase in energy, so you can increase your fuel-burning capacity and will feel more motivated to increase the exercise you need to make the dietary changes work. Bodies naturally plateau as they easily adapt to any new situation, so stick with it when weight loss seems to come to a halt; it will pick up again if you continue.

Sugar and Processed Foods

The more you look after what you do put into your body and prioritize the De-Stress lifestyle advice, the more you'll be able to easily and successfully handle tapering off sugars, stimulants and the sugar/fat combinations that your brain may have become used to receiving during stressful periods.[6] You'll realize by now that the most practical and useful tool here is to limit your insulin response to food and stress as our ancestors were doing naturally. In simple terms, it is stress and sugar that puts the weight around the middle. In order to regulate insulin and increase your nutrient, antioxidant and omega 3:6 oil ratios, increasing the good and reducing the bad makes every difference.

Avoid:

- **Processed fats low in omega 3 oils** – vegetable and seed oils (especially for cooking), poor quality spreads (use butter or olive oil), cheap refined oils, cheap meat and eggs, commercial mayonnaises and dressings.

- **Poor quality meat, eggs and fish** – unhealthy fats from sedentary, poorly fed animals that pass their bad luck on to you; processed meats like salami or those cured with nitrates. Pay more money and cut back on convenience or junk foods and things you don't need; with less stress you will find that comfort-buying lessens and you can redirect money to nourish you more.

- **Sugar and processed junk** – sugar in all its forms, sweeteners, damaged fats, ready-meals, take-away food ingredients that sound more like chemicals than food are just that.

Limit:

- **Grains/cereals** – wheat, rye, oats, barley flour, bran, quinoa, rice, corn, maize, all flours and 'milks' from these

- **Beans/legumes and pulses** – beans (soy, pinto, chickpea, mung, aduki, black, cannellini, etc.), peas, green beans, French beans, peanuts, ground nuts, pine nuts, flours like soy flour, gram flour, lentil flour in poppadoms, all flours and 'milks' from these

- **Roots that need cooking** – potatoes, sweet potatoes, parsnips, yams, cassava, tapioca

- **Dairy** – milk and skimmed milks, cheap cheese, fruit yoghurts (always sweetened) and processed powdered milk forms.

Finding a Balance

During the first phase of the De-Stress Diet plan, finding the right balance of grains, beans, starchy roots (such as potatoes and yams) and dairy can help insulin levels and appetite satisfaction.[7] For some people these foods can cause bloating, tiredness and indigestion as well as weight gain. For these people, cutting these foods out leads to effortless weight loss, an increase in energy and relief from a lifetime of post-lunch bloating. But for others, avoiding these starchy carbohydrates leaves them feeling listless, as though something is missing from their diets. During the first 3 weeks of this plan you will be able to decide if your individual chemistry responds best to a diet that includes small amounts of grains and beans cooked in the correct way. So, unless you're a vegetarian (and may need the protein from beans), during the first 3 weeks of this plan avoid grains and beans and take note of your energy levels. If you feel great and your stress symptoms, energy and weight improve, they may not suit you. If you find your energy levels lower, introduce one serving a day of beans at breakfast or lunch in the fourth week of this plan. In Chapter 6 you will find instructions for cooking your grains in safe and healthy ways.

• •

Troubleshooting: Weeks 1–3

PROBLEM: *Sugar cravings*

SOLUTION: First, too few fats or protein in your diet could be the answer; ensure you are including to satisfy your appetite.[8] Note any differences in sugar cravings without the presence of starches in your diet. Some may find they disappear altogether, others may find they crave sugar for energy. If you're in the latter group and really struggling, try a daily portion of either sourdough rye bread or soaked oats in the Bircher Muesli (page 90) at breakfast, or beans, new potatoes or a sweet potato at lunch for a few days. Experiment with these choices and if you still need help satisfying cravings as you move away from sugar, you may need a portion at both meals.

• •

PROBLEM: *Sugar cravings but bloating or inflammation from grain, beans and potatoes*

SOLUTION: Ensure you are eating plenty of dense vegetables such as broccoli, kale and asparagus, and include daily roots that can be eaten without cooking (but can also be cooked) like carrots, beetroot and radishes. Also ensure a daily piece of fruit and a portion of raw nuts and seeds.

- -

PROBLEM: *The urge to binge*

SOLUTION: Those who tend towards overeating or binge-eating can be set off by the insulin surge from grains, beans, potatoes, sweet potatoes, and of course refined sugars, stimulants and stress hormones. If you tend towards overeating or bingeing, cutting these out entirely may help reinstate the satiety hunger 'off switch'.

- -

PROBLEM: *Overeating nuts, seeds and dairy*

SOLUTION: Anecdotally, some overeaters may see bingeing episodes set off by eating too many nuts in a day. A palmful daily is enough for anyone (unless vegan) and if susceptible you may need less; seeds can be extra to the nut portion, but monitor their effects using the progress charts at the end of the book. The lactose in dairy may set off cravings, too.

Dairy and the 6-Week De-Stress Diet

Our ancestors didn't eat dairy but got their calcium (with magnesium) from green leaves, nuts and fish. In balance with plenty of weight-bearing exercise, this kept their bones strong. We advise avoiding dairy altogether if you can, or reducing your intake during the 6-Week Plan to an organic serving or two every 2–4 days.[9] If you are a vegetarian you may need to include a little more well-chosen dairy in your diet, ensuring probiotic levels are good to help you digest it.[10]

- **Greek feta cheese** from grass-fed goat's milk has a better fat profile than an average commercial cheddar or Swiss cheese. The feta has much lower saturated fat and contains omega 3 oils not found in cow's milk cheeses, making it healthier than a low-fat cheddar.[11]

- **Goat's and sheep's milk** products such as feta cheese are preferable as they contain smaller lactose (milk sugar) molecules and are easier for the gut to digest.

- **Greek yoghurt** contains less sugar and more protein than normal yoghurt, as it is sieved to remove the carbohydrate-rich whey. Its thickness leaves you fuller for longer (and you may need less) than more watery versions and the lower lactose – milk sugar – makes it easier to digest.

- **Hard cheese and butter** have lower lactose levels, so a lower insulin response than milk and cream. So, a slither or two of hard cheese every few days and a pat of butter on your vegetables are good choices, but remember that these are high in saturated fat so balance with other fats in olives, olive oil, nuts and seeds.

- **Whole-fat dairy** is preferable to skim milk, which is processed and less satisfying. Removing the fat strips away not just saturated fat, but also fat-soluble nutrients (important for lactose-tolerant vegetarians), the CLA that may help with weight loss (see page 52) and lots of healthy oleic acid (that in olive oil).

- **Farmer's produce** If you have access to a farm or farmers' market, buy raw milk and products legally directly from the farmer. This is milk that has not been pasteurized and therefore in its most natural state. There is evidence showing that this can have beneficial effects on the immune system and that there is less risk of bacterial contamination from animals better cared for in natural environments on the small farms that sell raw milk. If you are pregnant avoid these.

- **Avoid fruit yoghurts** These are an unnecessary source of added sugar. If you like a sweeter yoghurt, use plain wholemilk Greek yoghurt and add fresh fruit, coconut and cinnamon to sweeten and help balance blood sugar.

De-Stress Diet Supplements

We live in a world where all the nutrients we need are not always available in food because of poor soil and large-scale farming practices, and because the amounts we do absorb from food may be used up quickly by our bodies in response to stress, pollution and medications. If you are in the small minority reading this book from your log cabin on the side of a remote mountain, tending your flock and eating only from your naturally organic self-regulated ecosystem, the table below might not apply to you. For the rest of us, here is a basic supplement guide to help you make the most of the changes in the De-Stress 6-Week Plan. All of the below are safe to take long term and will aid your detoxification and energy levels during the first 6 weeks and beyond of your De-Stress Diet. We give you suggestions at de-stressyourlife.com,

Multivitamin and Mineral Supplement		
What –to include: B vitamins Chromium 400mcg Zinc 5–15mg Have with breakfast	**Sources** Pay for quality or you won't receive the right amount of nutrients in an absorbable form.	**Need to Know** Energy nutrients to support blood-sugar balance[12,13,14] Also shown to support weight-loss efforts[15,16,17]
Vitamin C		
1,000mg a day Avoid cheap, effervescent types with sweeteners added. Have with breakfast Optional extra with lunch if high stress, pollution, air travel or Stressed and Sore	**High amounts** strawberries, spring greens, blackcurrants, red peppers, watercress, oranges, lemons, kiwifruit **Moderate amounts** grapefruit, nectarines, bananas, spring onions, parsley, tomatoes, peaches, raspberries	Poor levels in modern food; helps absorb iron Higher need for this nutrient if under stress or exposed to pollution Naturally anti-inflammatory May help reduce cravings Supports liver detoxification[18,19]

Omega 3 oils – DHA and EPA

What

Only found in direct sources in fish oils, krill oil or algae (vegan source)

Fish oils: 2,000–4,000mg a day (usually 2–4 capsules) normal range with average of 325–330mg EPA/220–240mg DHA per 1,000mg

Krill oil: much less DHA and EPA but phospholipid form delivers to cells more easily

We recommend algae rather than plant sources for vegetarians as DHA/EPA needs to be converted from plant alpha-linoleic acid and believed to be only 5 per cent effective.

Sources

High amounts oily fish such as wild salmon, mackerel, trout, herring, sardines, anchovies

Plant sources walnuts, pumpkin seeds

Of all plant sources only flax has more omega 3 than 6 oils, but in a form that still needs converting, which can be compromised from stress and for those Stressed and Sore.

Need to Know

Modern diets are much higher in omega 6 oils and lower in omega 3 oils.

Appetite- and energy-regulating effects have been shown to support weight loss.[20,21]

May help reduce negative blood-sugar effects of stress[22]

Helps reduce the anxiety associated with psychological stress as well as mood and concentration, particularly krill oil[23,24,25,26]

Krill oil provides omega 3 oils from phospholipids which protect the brain from stress.[27]

Also available with vitamin D_3

Probiotics

Find a good-quality probiotic capsule or powder.

Main strains are lactobacillus and bifidobacteria, and others such as L. rhamnosus.

A good supplement has billions, not millions, of bacteria.

Probiotic yoghurts won't provide you with the human-strain organisms needed to repopulate your gut but they can help make the environment more conducive to colonizing these, alongside fermented foods and prebiotic soluble fibre (see list on page 31).

Those with better levels of beneficial, probiotic bacteria in their guts have shown to be able to break down phytic acid in grains and beans more efficiently.[28]

Low probiotic levels are linked to weight gain[29,30] and inflammation.

Stressed and Bloated Suits need to take a probiotic supplement, cut sugar down and eat more vegetables. This may be an important step for anyone keeping grains and beans in their diets.

Probiotics have shown to help reduce stress-related anxiety.[31]

Liver Support (optional)		
Milk thistle Artichoke Glutathione Turmeric	A dedicated liver-support tonic or supplement can help you through the changes but may release more toxins and produce more gas in the bowel to begin with so you might feel worse before you feel better.	Optimizing liver function has shown to help support weight loss programmes.[32] It may also help support the good digestion and blood-sugar balance that can help reduce sugar cravings and regulate appetite.
Adaptogenic Herb Support (optional)		
Rhodiola Gingko biloba Rehmannia Schisandra	Buy quality herbal supplements and follow instructions on the label building up from the lowest dose. Consult a qualified medical herbalist for specific advice.	These herbs work like a 'good stress', encouraging resistance and appropriate response to stressors via the brain.[33,34]

Weeks 1–3: Transition

In the first 3 weeks of the De-Stress Diet we focus on avoiding the following foods:

- **High-sugar/high-GI foods** – processed cereals, refined 'white' grains, soft drinks, fruit juices, added sugars, confectionery, sweets, chocolate, fruit 'flavoured' products, low-fat desserts including frozen yoghurt, alcohol

- **High-sugar/high-'bad' fat combination foods** – ice-cream, cakes, biscuits, pastries, cheap bread, pasties, sausage rolls, desserts with dairy and sugar, custard, cheap dark chocolate, any milk chocolate, commercial sandwiches

- **Gluten and dairy** – some people who have digestive and immune responses to the gluten in wheat, rye and barley (also oats if processed in the same factory as gluten-containing foods) and dairy may find that the chemical rush these might bring can set off sugar cravings, so worth avoiding fully for these 3 weeks. If you are a vegetarian, follow the healthy dairy guidelines above.

- **Stimulants** – alcohol, caffeine, nicotine, recreational drugs. If you have addictions to any of these, sorting out your sugar and stress issues first is the best preparation for giving them up, but you do need to be ready, so plan in this 6 weeks or give yourself a realistic goal for giving them up at a later date.

Recognizing and Accepting Addictions

Be kind to yourself during this phase. Regulating blood-sugar balance can take time after years of irregularities and you may initially have a period of adjustment where you crave sugar and refined foods more as your brain chemistry readjusts.[35] Sugar addiction fits four of the defined stages of addiction: bingeing, cravings, withdrawal and relapse,[36] and rats given the choice between sugar and cocaine overwhelmingly choose the sugar, even when the cocaine dose offered was raised.

Our first food, milk, was sweet, and then many of us were primed in childhood to see sugar as a source of 'comfort or reward'.[37] When we are stressed we can quickly revert to wanting[38]– and feeling we deserve – those comforting or rewarding feelings.[39] Changing this perception means accepting that these are only quick-fix solutions that ultimately rob us of sustained energy and a stable mood, while adding to weight gain. Use the De-Stress Progress Chart on pages 230–31 to help identify your own particular craving cycles.

Rebalancing

Pick a period to start this plan when you can have enough time and space to look after yourself such as a weekend where no one is coming to stay and you have free time to yourself. Remember, you're looking to make changes for life, not only to avoid things through gritted teeth for a short period of time. The supplement programme will help bring your body back to balance and supply nutrients commonly missing to help move you out of cravings cycles. As these positives increase, your need to rely on the negatives will decrease and more balanced biochemistry will take the place of willpower.

We all have blips in life, so if you don't live up to your ideal all the time, be kind to yourself and simply start again the next day. This is where the lifestyle advice can help, by buoying you up when your diet goes a little off the rails. Do the breathing calming techniques in Chapter 11 regularly to ensure you keep guilt and stress hormones down during this time. If you start beating yourself up, stop.

Possible Side Effects

Be prepared for sugar withdrawal effects such as headaches, irritability, anger, energy slumps, depression and fatigue.[40] You may also see signs that your detoxification processes and immune function are working, such as skin eruptions, phlegm or throat discomfort. For some people these can last weeks, but many people report feeling great once these initial symptoms have subsided. In women, you may also find one difficult menstrual cycle before monthly cycles and PMS improve.

Liver function is at the heart of balancing blood sugar and reducing cravings. Stress reduces the liver's ability to break down toxins and balance hormones, so lifestyle measures are crucial to managing these cycles on many levels. Every aspect of the De-Stress Diet helps improve detoxification and, alongside balancing gut bacteria and regulating brain function, we have seen many people go through a period where this release can lead to revisiting past emotions which they may feel they need to address. This is a time when you can see the powerful effect your diet and lifestyle has on your body and mind. Respect and accept how you're feeling, and use the Progress Chart on pages 230–31 to help the process.

Natural Detoxification

'Detox' does not refer just to a specialized cleansing ritual but is a natural process that occurs in every one of your cells, tissues and organs all the time. It is like breathing – as long as you are taking in air, water, food and substances from the environment, you will need to clear out the by-products. Getting waste products out of cells allows nutrients in, and relies on the right foods, less stress and circulation through movement, better breathing and fresh air.

You are likely to feel the effects of detoxification within these first few days to weeks. This will depend on your own liver capacity and previous habits. Don't be alarmed by any of the side effects described above; they're signs that you're making a positive difference and that there may be backed-up toxins circulating in your bloodstream – signs your liver needs more help. You can provide this help in these ways:

- **Hydration** Build up your pure water intake gradually especially if you have been underhydrated in the past (see page 151). Increase your herbal tea intake between meals and increase the amount of vegetables you eat.

- **Liver-supporting foods** See page 60 and try the suggestions on page 81.

- **Circulation** Keep circulation moving with short outdoor walks, gentle yoga (especially Viparita Karani – see page 221), lying-down or seated twists and breathing exercises as described in Chapter 11, even embracing the cold shower for a few seconds.

- **Massage, saunas and steams** Will help calm your nerves, lower stress hormones and release toxins in muscles and through skin.

- **Dry skin-brushing** This is the perfect De-Stress self-care ritual, with friction from the dry brush bristles increasing circulation and drawing toxins out towards the skin. Buy a not-too-soft body brush with all natural bristles and, once a day before a bath or shower, brush in long strokes all over your body towards the heart.

- **Ayurvedic oils** After a bath or shower, before drying, quickly rub unrefined organic sesame or linseed oil straight onto your skin. This is an ancient Ayurvedic practice that helps promote circulation and detoxification.

- **Epsom salts baths** Use a cupful (from pharmacies) to help both release tight muscles (including the bowel) and to detoxify. Stay for

20 minutes but don't have it too hot (the brave can have a cold shower afterwards for a thermogenic sauna/spritz effect).

Keep on Moving

A daily bowel movement is crucial for eliminating the day's toxins and metabolic wastes, but also regulating hormones, cholesterol and immunity. If you experience constipation, follow the previous liver-support advice, increasing soluble fibre through vegetables, nuts and fruit and ensuring good bowel hydration with the measures on page 81. In addition you can:

- **Relax** Some people find simply reading a book on the loo helps them relax and gets things moving.

- **Exercise** Squatting motions and abdominal exercises stimulate peristalsis, the movement of muscles in the gut. These muscles need daily toning as much as any other.

- **Practise yoga breathing and postures** Can help the gut relax – especially twists, which massage the intestines.

- **Take magnesium supplements** (page 127) These can help release spasm or seizure in gut muscles which can lead either to constipation or diarrhoea.

- **Try Bircher Muesli** (page 90) with extra prunes and/or unsulphured dried apricots soaked and added in, or with added stewed plums, apples and soaked linseeds, will have a natural laxative effect.

- **Drink aloe vera juice** Can help constipation,[41] but do not take it for longer than 3 months at a time or the bowel can start to rely on it. Take as directed – up to a quart a day of juice or 2 tablespoons pure gel on an empty stomach. Or add it to fruit juice or peppermint tea before bed and on rising. Aloe juice can also be taken with turmeric or crushed fennel seeds to prevent tummy pains; some herbalists recommend taking it for 5 days, stopping for 2, then starting again for 3 months maximum to prevent allergic build-up.

Realistic, Steady, Lifelong Change

From sugary snacks to pizza, the fewer of your 'habit foods' you have, the easier it gets and you will soon see that your tastes change. It can take just days for a sweet tooth to decrease and for sugary foods to start to taste overly so. So stick with it and the foods you may think you can't live without may suddenly seem less appealing. We advise three meals a day and no snacks in the De-Stress Diet; the right meal at the right time should be able to sustain blood sugar for the 4–5 hours until the next, and allow for full digestion and natural signs of mild hunger in between. However, for those with long-term blood-sugar issues, the right snack at the right time can help curb cravings for sugar at other times. See Chapter 9 for snack suggestions.

Retraining Your Taste Buds

Sugar, salt and chemical flavourings can numb taste buds so that sub-tle tastes such as those of herbs and vegetables seem less appealing. These substances also alter brain chemistry and the way we respond to foodstuffs. During these 3 weeks you will be changing your palate and tasting more subtle and sophisticated flavours so that you begin to enjoy healthier foods.

Sugar-craving Solutions

Giving up sugar 'cold turkey' can initially lead to poor glucose supply to the brain, which causes poor serotonin regulation and a subsequent drop in mood. This can happen about 3–4 days after giving up sugar, and can lead to binges and cravings. Again this is temporary as your system gets used to slower-release forms of fuel to the body and brain.

Use the De-Stress sugar weaning tips on page 147, together with the following suggestions to help you make lasting changes:

- We typically have a blood-sugar low around 4 p.m. when traditionally the tea and cakes were wheeled out. If this is your time of least resistance, eat a healthy snack at this time or just before. Although less snacking is the ideal scenario, it is preferable to choose a better snack at the right time than mainline the sugar later. See Chapter 9 for suggestions.

- Constant cravings for sugar can indicate that there are not enough healthy, quality proteins and fats in your diet.[42] Be particularly aware of this if you are vegetarian or (especially) a vegan.

- Choose fruits such as apples, berries or plums over less tart fruits if you have a sweet tooth. These have been shown to reduce sugar spikes after meals.[43,44]

- Xylitol is the best sugar substitute choice, with some positive effects seen on weight loss, but it can keep a sweet tooth alive.[45] Substitute it for sugar in tea or coffee, then wean yourself off it bit by bit over a few weeks.

- Use sweet tastes that don't upset blood-sugar. These include unsweetened coconut, ground almond, natural vanilla essence and unsweetened apple puree. Coconut provides a natural sweetness and contains plant-saturated fats called medium-chain triglycerides (MCTs) that help satisfy any needs for sugar as they provide a dense energy source. Use as unsweetened desiccated coconut or flakes.

- Use cinnamon as much as possible; it contains a bioflavonoid called MHCP that mimics insulin, actively moving sugar into cells for energy and sensitizing insulin receptors.[46] A teaspoon a day helps balance blood-sugar levels in people with diabetes. It is highly effective at telling the brain that you have eaten something sweet with positive rather than negative consequences. Add to coffee, tea, yoghurt, berries, curries. (Also see the list of spice teas on page 152.)

- An effective Ayurvedic (Indian traditional medicine) trick to curb cravings is an eggcup full of aloe vera juice with a pinch each of cinnamon and turmeric between meals. This may also help ease constipation.

- A small portion of starchy carbs such as new potatoes or sweet potatoes can be included at dinner if you are suffering late-night binges. You can then wean yourself off this as you regulate energy and cravings while giving up refined sugars.[47]

- You may feel you want to give up caffeine in the pursuit of your De-Stress aims, but if you have a bit of a sugar or refined carbo-hydrate habit to give up at this time, wait or just cut back. Giving up sugar and caffeine at the same time can knock your energy for six, especially if you wear a Stressed and Tired Suit. The sugar issue is far more important than one or two cups of caffeine with food (see pages 152–56). Try licorice tea to substitute a natural lift but, as with caffeine, it is best avoided after mid-afternoon or it may affect sleep.

- If you are suffering mood dips or energy lows, use the calming and breathing techniques in Chapter 11 to come down from the exacerbating stress response these feelings might bring.

Weeks 4–6: True Change

By now you will have an understanding of how the food you choose and the lifestyle choices you make affect way you feel and look. Not because we say so, but through personal experience. This 'sense mem-ory' and intuition are more powerful than anything we can say.[48] It's likely you will also be moving your life to a more balanced place as the nutrition, relaxation and lifestyle practices have an impact on your weight, stress levels and mood. For some people this can take longer as they settle into new ways of shopping and understanding healthy food choices and cooking, but it is an enjoyable and illuminating journey. You have the chance to learn more about yourself than we could ever tell you, as there are emotional and physical implications within the different minutiae of everybody's lives and these will become apparent as you make these changes. This can bring you more mental and emotional clarity if you stay mindful, and help you identify areas of your life where bigger changes may need to be made. Hopefully, you will soon have the energy and clarity to make these.

For these 3 weeks, continue to follow the guidelines outlined at the beginning of this chapter and using the De-Stress Diet Every Day chapters to put these into practice. This will help you stay connected to your new, more refined taste buds. The main change during these 3 weeks is that during this time you have the option to introduce occasional treats such as a little bit of alcohol or chocolate to your diet. Unrealistic and over-regimented diets never work long term, and so these 3 weeks are about setting the scene for true change and deciding what will work for you on a daily and weekly basis. Stay flexible so you don't promote the stress cycles of setting yourself up to fail or beating yourself up about the odd treat. The most important part of the De-Stress Diet is allowing change to settle and take effect, and these 3 weeks are about observing how the changes make you feel, what works for you and what you will take with you into the rest of your life.

A Bean/Grain Plan

By now you've worked out whether cutting out grains and beans entirely works for you or whether 1–2 servings a day suits you better. If you choose to include wholegrains and beans, avoid them at dinner to increase the likelihood that your level of activity over the rest of the day will regulate the fat-storing potential of the insulin they cause to be released.

If you are a vegetarian, stick to one serving of grains and one of beans, but not at the same meal. Or serve a half-portion of each only. Beans are easier to include safely, as the correct cooking processes can break down phytic acid more readily (see Chapter 6).

For most non-vegetarians, one portion of grains and/or beans maximum daily is ample, especially if far outweighed by vegetables, good protein and healthy fats in your diet.

During the next 3 weeks, revisit the Troubleshooting suggestions on pages 63–64 and explore the following options:

- **If you want to lose weight:** Replace grains, beans and potatoes with vegetables, nuts and seeds. Remember that these are still carbohydrate plant foods, but have more soluble than insoluble fibre for greater appetite control. A recent study showed that with only a 10g daily increase in soluble fibre, 3.7 per cent of dangerous deep belly fat was reduced over five years.[49] This is worth exploring if you are Stressed and Bloated or Stressed and Sore.

- **If you have been eating some grains, beans or potatoes to help with sugar withdrawal:** You may now be in a place to explore removing them to monitor craving or binge cycles.

- **If you want to include beans/grains and are vegetarian or vegan:** Your best choice is a slice of sourdough rye bread or soaked oats in the Bircher Muesli (see page 90) at breakfast or a small portion of well-cooked beans, new potatoes or sweet potato at lunch. Always eat with vegetables that provide vitamin C to help reduce anti-nutrients and absorb iron.

- **If you experience constipation:** This might result from reducing the amount of insoluble fibre you'd normally get from grains and beans, even while increasing soluble fibre levels in vegetables, fruit and nuts. See the 'Keep on Moving' section of this chapter (pages 71 and 81). If this doesn't improve things in a fortnight, add 1–2 daily portions of whole grains and beans.

Healthy Grain Guidelines

If you decide to include grains in your diet, avoid cheap, commercial breads and choose instead small bakery and sourdough loaves. Also avoid raw grains in mueslis and unfermented soy in soy milk and flour. Switch to rye where possible, as this contains less gluten than wheat and more phytase, the enzyme that breaks down phytic acid (Chapter 5) and helps iron and zinc absorption.[50] Sourdough rye bread is the best choice, as the fermentation with lactic acid breaks this down even more.[51] Rye also naturally contains lactic acid to help break down anti-nutrients – this is why soaking oats in lactic acid containing yoghurt for the Bircher muesli is the best cereal choice. Avoid wheat to give your digestion and immune system a break from the high gluten content. Even if you're not intolerant this will help your beneficial gut bacteria, and this may positively impact your serotonin levels and mood.

Find your personal grain tolerance levels by avoiding foods you find you react to (with bloating, discomfort or tiredness). This is the ideal, at any rate, but not always possible, so simply keep your intake minimum or occasional. You may see that you can handle fewer grains and beans when you're stressed – often, ironically, the times when you're not able to make the best choices (for example, that dodgy sandwich at the airport after a long-haul flight). The more you can help yourself with better choices when they're available, the less you will react to the exceptions.

Treats and Habits – Learning the Difference

If blood-sugar balance is regulated our bodies can handle the odd spike. To achieve this you need to be clear about the difference between a treat and a habit.

Treat: an occasional enjoyment of something that gives you pleasure but that you do not feel controlled by; yes, you deserve it occasionally, but you are aware that ultimately it works against your health and weight.

Habit: something you eat habitually – that is, regularly, every day or every few days.

If eating a food you consider to be a treat makes you feel guilty or as if you are failing, ask yourself whether it is creeping in as a habit or if you are being too hard on yourself.

Experiment

It can be easier when you have a strict no-go policy on the so-called 'baddies', but this can become another source of psycho-social stress for those who don't like rules or authority. Observe your reactions from the first 3 weeks. If complete avoidance of the odd treat works for you, identify and accept that. If you need to know you can have that indulgence two or three times a week or you'll rebel and eat the whole cake shop, know that too and plan the right way to do it. One of the authors of this book has fish and chips once a month without fail and it deeply satisfies any want for that giddy carb/fat combination she might otherwise succumb to at other times.

Quality Not Quantity

Pick your treats based on quality, not quantity. For example, a few quality chocolate Brazil nuts rather than a large bar of a more processed, sugary kind. Higher-quality foods like this are often more satisfying; what is the point of a treat that you don't fully enjoy? Or if wine is your treat, a better-quality wine and half as much can help you savour it. Stop before you hit the point where you feel unhealthy or guilty, and find the point where you can control cravings but not deny yourself, so you don't feel the need to rebel but are still getting results, enjoying yourself and moving away from feeling confused or neurotic around food. Other examples of quality treats include a 40g block of organic 70 per cent dark chocolate, a small cup of high-quality gourmet ice-cream or a small serving of homemade pudding. You get the idea.

Addictions

If you have addictive patterns to other substances such as caffeine beyond a couple of cups a day, alcohol, cigarettes or recreational drugs, consider at what stage you now see yourself without the influence of chronic stress, sugar, refined carbohydrates and excess junk fats. Be careful not to increase your intake of these to replace sugar[52] so that from there you can plan when you might feel the right time to give up. Continuing with the De-Stress Diet and lifestyle tools will help you create the energy and brain chemicals that will make giving up these other things far easier.

Your De-Stress Journal

This is a period when you can take stock and record what works best for you and what doesn't. Use the reflective practice below to help you start a personal De-Stress journal. Ask yourself these questions at least once a week, ideally more often, and jot down the answers in your journal. You can keep coming back to the questions to help you reflect on how your De-Stress lifestyle is making you feel, function and look, and to identify any tweaks or changes you need to make.

1. Are you feeling more connected to your body and intuition around food, stress and your day-to-day needs? Have you identified where you might tend to 'push on through' despite your body's obvious cries for rest, care and support?

2. Are sweet foods tasting too sweet? Are you enjoying the more subtle tastes of good-quality produce and flavourings?

3. Note how different days require different approaches. Are you now learning to be adaptable and respect your body's altering needs, rather than expecting one strategy to work every single day? Have you noticed any particular eating/energy patterns over 3- or 4-day cycles?

4. Do you feel you have started on a journey and may need to do further tests with a nutritional therapist for things such as food intolerance, thyroid function or adrenal stress profile? Go back to the Stress Suits chapter and see if your symptoms have improved. If they still feel entrenched you may need to seek out more specific attention. At de-stressyourlife.com you will find the resources and help you need.

5. Variety is key, so don't settle into new fixed regimens – our ancestors ate hundreds more foods than we do and these changed with the seasons, limiting the likelihood of food intolerance and provid-

ing the right nutrient balance for the climate. Have you found ways to vary your food content to ensure your shopping and cooking are rewarding and done mindfully rather than on auto-pilot?

6. Assess your relationship with grains and beans – will it work best for you to include some occasionally or are you feeling so good that you want to continue to mainly avoid them?.

7. Too much of anything – partying, working, parenting – without the requisite balance of recharging and self-care will always wear you down. Are there any areas of your life where you still see yourself creating unnecessary stress? What kind of limits could you place on yourself to free yourself up for other pursuits that calm or energize you?

8. Has the way you cope with stress changed? Think about any habitual reactions such as overeating, sugar cravings or flying off the handle that you might have experienced when stress hit before you began 3 weeks ago. When was the last time this happened and how did you cope? In terms of De-Stress Diet lifestyle measures, which work best for you? Are you managing to bring breathing techniques, mindfulness and meditation in simple ways into your life to help relieve stress on a daily basis? A few minutes is all it takes.

Further Detox

If you would like extra self-care or you are still seeing symptoms of detoxification like headaches or bloating, or are feeling sluggish or constipated, try the following to optimize your detoxification capacity:

Start each morning with a *liver flush* – juice of one grapefruit and one lemon, 2 tablespoons extra-virgin olive oil, 1 crushed clove garlic, 1 inch ginger root, grated – mix and drink down 15 minutes before breakfast. This can be done for just 1 week for good results. Mix the night before and keep in the fridge.

Consider using sunflower (or soy) lecithin to break down fats in the liver, especially if you are a vegan, as this is your only source of the B vitamin choline.

Rub unrefined organic sesame or linseed oil into your entire body before your bath or shower (after dry brushing). Make this a thoroughly relaxing experience by lying for 20 minutes in (slippery) Savasana (page 221) to allow it to soak in.

Exercise is a key part of liver detoxification, specifically strong calves and thighs with good upper body posture. This combination ensures strong circulation around the liver and a full oxygen and nutrient supply to keep it happy.

Reviewing Your Progress

You might want to revisit any of the following to give yourself some perspective on where you are and where you are heading. After all, you are unravelling years of stressful living and are just at the beginning. You can use what follows to do your own self-assessment, identifying the times when you may need to use the tools you have discovered to guide you back if previous habits sneak in:

- The Stress Quiz on page xi

- The Stress Suits Quiz starting on page 19

- De-Stress Journal on page 80

- De-Stress Progress Charts on pages 223–31

See de-stressyourlife.com to download these and others for repeated use.

6-Week Plan Support

Let us know the day you are starting The De-Stress Diet at de-stressyourlife.com and we will send you supporting emails and weekly De-Stress Expert Support podcasts with extra motivation and well-timed tips along your journey.

Chapter 5

A BREAKFAST REVOLUTION

One of the most profound things you can do for your health is to start your day well. Breakfast is the meal that can either set up your good mood, energy and coping capacity for the coming day or set you off on a giddy ride of bouncing between craving quick fixes and struggling for motivation. The right meal after the long period without food overnight can have the greatest knock-on effect on your food choices throughout the day. Eat well when you wake up and you reinforce your ability to choose healthier foods because you are not at the whim of disordered biochemistry. In other words, the right breakfast in the morning means few cravings later. We can't overstate this: those 4 p.m. and late-night sweet or crisp cravings can be traced back to the wrong input at the start of your day. Your body is intelligent – feed it incorrectly in the morning and it will play a nasty game of energy 'catch-up' with you all day in the form of cravings and mood swings.

You probably already know how a good breakfast makes sense, but until you've experienced the effects it can have on your body the habit won't stick. Habits are created out of rich 'sense memories' and these are based on your experienced senses and feelings, so you won't create a true paradigm shift, a new way of living, without finding a nourishing, robust and satisfying morning habit that works for you. This chapter will help you find that. Work with the suggestions until you find what nourishes you and gives you the best start to every day.

Most Important Meal of the Day

Nutrition experts may have differing opinions on many things, but the need for breakfast is not one of them. Skipping breakfast has shown to cause weight, focus, mood and appetite problems.[1,2] Our metabolism is designed to take in most calories at the beginning half of each day to fuel the search for more food. Protein for breakfast, in particular, has been shown to satisfy appetite for longer than a high-carb breakfast (like cereal),[3] and fats included for breakfast show better results in the level of morning blood-sugar balance than the low-fat options.[4] Many people who struggle to lose weight eat little for breakfast and lunch and pile up the calories – often as refined carbs – towards the end of the day when digestion and metabolism have slowed right down, making these calories more likely to be laid down as fat. Skipping breakfast in an attempt to lose weight will backfire,[5] as it tends to result in poor food choices throughout the day. If you don't fuel up on rising, stress hormones such as adrenaline and cortisol take over to raise blood-sugar levels. Skipping any meal translates as prolonged fasting, a state that can raise your body's insulin response and therefore fat storage and weight gain, especially around the middle.

Breakfast as a Meal

Breakfast has become more about convenience and less about choice, care and mindfulness. Our morning routines are yet another casualty of our over-subscribed diaries, leaving it less of a meal – with variety and enjoyment – and more a glorified snack. Many people feel they are at least eating healthily at this meal, but tea and toast or boxed cereals are more comfort foods than healthy breakfast foods.

'I Don't Have Time'

You may assume that making changes to this part of your day might create more stress. After all, you're far too tired and rushed to make *more* time first thing – can't you just make up for it the rest of the day? It may seem hard to imagine now, but there will come a time when you look forward to your day-break ceremony because it increases your effectiveness throughout the day. What you do in the morning vastly influences your food choices, energy levels and ability to cope with life's challenges throughout the day. This means better quality sleep and, therefore, waking refreshed the next day.

By waking smoothly and taking just a bit of time to prepare yourself for the day's demands, you can give yourself space to taste and enjoy food that is good for digestion and appetite-regulation; sustaining food rescues you from frustrating and exhausting daytime highs and lows. It's feeling good – not willpower – that stops us turning to junk food and overeating. The De-Stress Diet is about breaking vicious cycles, and breakfast is our most important tool for this.

Think Outside the (Cereal) Box

Look at habits across the world and you'll notice that foods we consider breakfast fare in the West come from a fairly small range of choices. People eat grilled fish and vegetables in Korea, fish and coconut *sambol* in Sri Lanka, dim sum in some Thai provinces and meats, smoked fish and cheeses in Scandinavian countries – choices that are more nutritionally supportive than the glut of processed grain products such as cereals and breads most of us eat. It's no coincidence that the typical Western breakfast of boxed cereal, white bread and high-sugar jam has soared in popularity alongside the rise of obesity, diabetes and heart disease.

The De-Stress Diet bottom-line breakfast rule is simple: *eat healthy food you enjoy*. Don't feel that you have to force down that porridge or muesli because 'it's good for me'. Experiment with freeing yourself from the herd, try our suggestions and monitor how your mind and body respond. You might be surprised.

Variety Matters

Breakfast is a meal like any other and you can get bored and miss out on the full range of nutrients if you get stuck in a rut. Feel free to vary as you choose and experiment from the options below, or make up your own based on the guidelines on pages 87–88. You can eat anything at breakfast, even last night's left-over curry (Charlotte's favourite), or Anna's go-to special when home in Australia: fresh king prawns, oysters and a ripe, local mango. All of the dinner and lunch suggestions in coming chapters make great breakfasts and are an easy way to prepare food in advance.

Wake-up Call

For the die-hard 'don't eat 'til 11a.m.' types, consider this period of waking up your morning metabolism your new project for Phase 1, the 3-week transitional plan.

Start the day with the juice of half a lemon in hot water to wake up your liver and digestion in a clean, healthy way. Drink this about 20 minutes before breakfast – you can also add slices of fresh ginger to warm up or calm the digestion, and/or cinnamon to sweeten and improve blood-sugar balance.

DSD Tip

If you're used to having a cup of coffee or tea before breakfast, save this until you have food in your stomach. If you drink coffee or tea when blood-sugar levels are low, you'll get a surge as your body produces adrenaline in response to the caffeine and won't feel the need of food to raise them.

Breakfast Like a King

What	Why	How
This creates a positive effect on appetite and cravings, and helps level out mid-afternoon energy dips and late-night binges that cause weight gain.	Reclaiming breakfast time sets up our body rhythms in the way they've evolved to work. We are designed to use the calories we get in the morning to move around rather than laying them down as fat when we sleep.	Experiment with breakfast suggestions on pages 88–90. Always have something. If you're buying out, look for some protein and always keep some raw, unsalted nuts in your bag just in case. If you're always on the run, check out our snack bar guide on page 147 to stock up on easy cupboard breakfast emergencies. Prepare to eat, by taking ten full, natural breaths before starting.
Protein for breakfast	Satisfies appetite for longer, raises metabolism, keeps insulin production low and reduces fat-storing tendencies.	Animal proteins like meat, fish, eggs or dairy provide complete protein – all the amino acid building-blocks we need to help build muscle. Eggs have been shown time and again to help weight loss when eaten at breakfast as the filling choice that creates better glucose/insulin response and food choices for the rest of the day[6,7] and have been shown to help weight loss.[8] Nuts and seeds (and their butters) are among the most natural proteins and starchy foods we can eat, also providing fats and healthy omega oils; our ancestors were eating them long before we starting growing grains and pulses. Keep nut butters like hazelnut and pumpkin seed in the fridge for a quick protein addition to rye bread or crackers. Note that peanuts are a bean, not a nut, and can cause inflammation. For vegans, including beans and pulses for breakfast can be an important protein to help cope with the day's stress; try the stews on page 102 for breakfast to ensure most phytic acid is broken down and most digestible.

Complex Carbohydrates First Thing		
Fuel the brain and muscles immediately.	The best fuel comes not only from starches like bread and cereal, but also from other complex carbohydrate in whole plant sources such as nuts, seeds, fruit, vegetables.	Best-case scenario is using breakfast as another opportunity to get in a vegetable portion: avocados, watercress, tomatoes, spinach all make perfect breakfast foods (yes, we know avocado is technically a fruit...). Fruit is best as an energy source when kept intact and not with fibre removed as a juice, so have your fruits whole, not juiced. Nuts provide starches alongside protein and fat, and are perfect nutritional parcels – add to porridge or cereal soaked overnight for digestibility.

De-Stress Breakfast – Three Options to Explore

Use the De-Stress Progress Chart – Energy, Mood and Appetite on pages 230–31 to compare how different combinations make you feel in terms of cravings, 'highs and lows' and appetite.

1. Breakfast Outside the Box

The best basis for starting the day, especially if you tend to have sugar cravings, can be prepared the night before as you make dinner.

Choose from a protein source:

- Eggs – 1–2 boiled, poached, omelet or slowly scrambled

- Fish – smoked mackerel, trout or salmon fillet cooked night before

- Goat's or sheep's cheese – e. g. feta or soft cheese

- 2 turkey or chicken slices

- (Occasionally) good-quality sausages, ham or bacon

- Portion prepared beans or nut burger if vegan

Add a portion (palm-sized) of at least 2 of the following:

- Avocado
- Tomatoes

- Asparagus
- Spinach
- Watercress
- Cucumber

- Cooked beetroot (not in vinegar)
- Rocket
- Artichokes
- or any other veg

2. The Healthy 'British'

A good 'grounding' breakfast for the recovering sugar junkie:

- Poached, slow-scrambled eggs or omelet

- Good-quality free-range bacon (2 slices) or sausage (1–2 depending on size), grilled – just once or twice a week total as contain nitrate preservatives (unless you can buy without). Alternatively, a high-quality lamb or beefburger is a nitrate-free occasional option. For a vegetarian or different protein option, either grill 2 Portobello mushrooms (with olive oil), grill some halloumi or grill 2 good-quality nut burgers instead.

- 2 halves of a medium tomato, grilled, or 4–6 cherry tomatoes oven roasted with a little olive oil.

- Optional vegetable portion: wilted spinach or asparagus

- Add a third of a tin of baked beans – choose low sugar or a brand sweetened with apple juice (such as Whole Earth) from a health food shop.

DSD Tip

If you find you are better suited to a small portion of starchy carb with your savoury breakfast, buy more expensive quality breads. Loaves can be sliced and frozen to pull out individual portions to toast. Sourdough rye is better digested and evidence suggests rye bread may boost feelings of fullness when eaten at breakfast. Eat with butter, nut butters or olive oil and avoid hydrogenated or high-sunflower oil spreads.

3. Bircher Muesli Medley

This is the best alternative to muesli if you want a morning starchy carb, as the oats and nuts are soaked and so easier to digest and lower in phytic acid:

- Soak 35g (about 2 tablespoonfuls) rolled oats in yoghurt or alternatively water or half-water/half-freshly pressed apple juice overnight in the fridge with a tablespoon of nuts and seeds for protein – choose from almonds, Brazils, walnuts, pecans, sunflower and pumpkin seeds. You can add a dessertspoon of golden linseeds for increased detoxifying, digestive and hormonal health if you want.

- Sweeten only with ground cinnamon, unsweetened desiccated coconut and fruit from these options: chopped dried apricots, prunes, grated apple, berries, sliced or stewed plums and/or apples.

- For variety or a gluten-free option, buckwheat, quinoa or millet flakes can be used in place of oats, or mixed in with them.

- You can add a dollop of plain live Greek or live plain wholemilk yoghurt to taste if the oats have been soaked in water/apple juice.

- For speed, mix up your grains, nuts and seeds and keep in an airtight container to quickly pour into a bowl.

How You Have Breakfast

Nourishing yourself isn't only about what you eat, but how you eat it. Here's the ideal De-Stress morning routine, with options depending on the time you have. Taking any of the attitudes on board is a positive move and will impact your stress levels and mood throughout the day.

Your Stress-free Morning

- Wake up and give yourself time (even just 30 seconds) before leaping into action; then ease out of bed by standing up slowly. This tells your body there is no imminent danger. Have a stretch.

- Drink some lemon juice with hot water and optional cinnamon and ginger.

- This may be a good time for a walk, meditation, breathing exercise or morning yoga sequence: yoga postures or other stretching are best done before food so digestion doesn't steal energy from your muscles. Set a soft alarm for the time allotted so no panic sets in. Experiment with the time and your choice of exercise to feel relaxed. It can take time to find what's right for you. Don't feel you have to spend the same time every morning. If you miss one, just start again the next day.

- Prepare breakfast. Do you faff about or get sidetracked by other things? Stick to the task and feel like this is an important part of self-care. Make the process as simple as possible: prepare some things the night before, try to keep the kitchen clean and organized.

- Don't start bolting your food standing up or take it with you to get ready; sit at a table and place it in front of you, then take the 10 Deep Breaths exercise (see page 195) to prepare for digestion.

- Eat breakfast. Eat calmly and take at least 15 minutes, chewing every mouthful and actually tasting your food. If you eat slowly enough and chew well, you should naturally allow digestion to happen more easily. Include sitting for 5 minutes after you have finished eating as part of your breakfast time.

- Enjoy what you eat. If you don't enjoy your meal, make changes the next day but bear in mind if you're missing a sweeter breakfast it can take a few days for your taste buds to change.

- Ease into your day. If you're not taking time for breathing, meditation, etc. after breakfast (see below), it can seem a tall order not to jump to action after eating, but anything you can do to keep yourself from becoming stressed can help your food go down. This can ensure full digestion of nutrients to make you feel fuller and keep you sated until lunchtime.

Those Stressy Habits Resolved

- If waking is difficult see the sleep solutions on pages 124–25. You may want to do a simple breathing exercise before getting out of bed, see page 195.

- If worries are taking you out of the present moment, it may help to write them down now or the night before to put them to rest.

- If you are used to running out of the door as soon as you've stuffed in breakfast, it can really reclaim the day to take a pause before you go.

- If you have only 2–10 minutes for an exercise routine, try the Morning Priority yoga poses or breathing session from Chapter 11.

- If you have more time (15–20 minutes), try the Full Morning Yoga Sequence (page 209), a stroll around the block or a short jog if you are an exercise bunny, but not to the point of feeling adrenaline kicking in – this is individual but you'll know it by your heart suddenly racing.

- Prepare as much as you can for the morning the night before: clothes, bath and things you need for your day.

- If you leave for work, leave with a smile. If you work from home, separate your working environment from your morning preparation, even go for a walk around the block as if you are 'going to work'. If it's a weekend, factor in time at least one day to rest for an hour or two after breakfast to properly recharge from the week.

Making the Transition Work for You

Like Rome, a De-Stress Diet and lifestyle wasn't built in a day. Here are some suggestions to help see you through the shift from your current routine to De-Stress success. Remember, every small step towards change counts.

Stressy Start	Finding Your Balance	De-Stress Success
Nothing for breakfast!	Take 10 deep breaths (see page 195) and then at least have a small version of a breakfast, a snack option or even a few nuts and half an apple – anything is better than nothing. If you really don't want to eat, make a quick coconut milk and berry smoothie (you can take the berries straight from the freezer and blend).	Build up to at least a calmly eaten smaller breakfast in the week and more at the weekend. This tells your body it is not in a famine and does not need to slow down metabolism or store fat.
Processed cereal and a coffee	A smaller version of Bircher Muesli Medley (see page 90) or even a granola-type cereal with the same amount of nuts and seeds.	Bircher Muesli Medley or Breakfast Outside the Box (see page 85) whenever possible. If you can curb the rush and get up 10–15 minutes earlier (because your sleep quality will improve), decide your morning calming activity before bed and prepare a space.
Fairly good breakfast, but 1 or 2 hours after waking	Any movement towards closer to when you get up is progress. Explore how you feel as you move this to a calmer state.	Move breakfast to 15–20 minutes after rising and make space to prioritize your morning routine.
Bolting food in between feeding the kids, dog and husband	Watch where this is being put upon you and where you are letting it happen. Remember, if you don't make even a little space for yourself (just 10 breaths?), you'll eventually run out of energy to look after other people.	Achieve days where you are looked after or even have the kids looked after – even once a week or every fortnight can make a difference. Eat with the kids to encourage them to be more mindful and therefore create space for you; they can eat the same as you, or versions of it.

· ·

Troubleshooting: Breakfast

PROBLEM: *You get a 6.30 a.m. train or have a long drive to work and then eat at your desk.*

SOLUTION: Take 10 deep breaths before eating and chew thoroughly and calmly. Prioritize breakfast before work or pack a smoothie with coconut milk and berries. If you have your breakfast on the train or at your desk, focus on that with no work or phone calls at the same time. Try soup, stew or porridge in a flask for the colder months. Good-quality containers and food-carrying bags make transportation easy. Keep nut butters to add to sourdough rye or crackers, suggested snack bars on page 147 and nuts for days when you have less time. Download meditations, visualizations or music you find soothing to listen to on your journey.

. . . .

PROBLEM: *You go to the gym before work and never know what to eat.*

SOLUTION: Time to get ready, go to the gym and then work out can mean not eating for a few hours after getting up. This is not advised, especially with intense exercise where stress hormones are raised. Have a smoothie with coconut milk and berries before, and then your full breakfast straight after. Add some whey protein to your pre-workout smoothie to support blood-sugar levels during longer sessions. Ensure your workouts are varied and not adding to your stress levels (see Chapter 10).

. . . .

PROBLEM: *You can't see an improvement in your energy.*

SOLUTION: Check the Stressed and Tired recommendations – including iron and vitamin B_{12} – and consider taking a co-enzyme Q10 supplement (see opposite).

Focus on Co-enzyme Q10 (aka Co-Q10 or ubiquinone)

Normal supplementation range: 30–200mg daily Best forms: fat-soluble capsules or liquid	Food sources: poultry, beef, broccoli, mackerel, organ meats, sardines, spinach, soy	What it does: Transforms food into ATP, the body's energy fuel, helping you move on from reliance on sugar and stimulants for energy. The body can make Co-Q10 but it relies on selenium and levels naturally drop as we get older.[10,11,12]

Help by Stress Suit

	You may find that you...	Best single change you could make
Stressed and Wired	start the day in a frenzy of stress hormones	Make time to do a full 15-minute calming activity to retrain your nervous system.
Stressed and Tired	drag yourself to vertical and really don't want to get out of bed	Have a protein breakfast and chew thoroughly; make at least a little time to build up energy through full breathing.
Stressed and Cold	feel sluggish and heavy as you haul yourself upright	Get moving slowly and stretch to get your circulation going; include ginger in your morning hot lemon.
Stressed and Bloated	feel uncomfortable first thing and have an unsatisfactory bowel movement or none when you want one	Have lemon in hot water to stimulate liver and pancreas function; consider digestive enzymes with breakfast, and chew!
Stressed and Sore	wake feeling heady, itchy or phlegmy	Choose the activity that most calms you to stop setting off inflammatory reactions that might show up as achy joints, skin, digestive or nasal issues or headaches.
Stressed and Demotivated	feel no joy or downright dread the coming day	Choose a meditation or breathing exercise that works for you to do sitting up in bed. Ensure protein and B vitamins for brain chemical action.
Stressed and Hormonal	wake irritable and tetchy	Include liver-supporting foods for breakfast such as smoked salmon or mackerel, nuts, seeds, avocado, beetroot and watercress.

Chapter 6

THE BUILDING BLOCKS OF LUNCH AND DINNER

There's no hidden secret to healthy cooking. Once you know a few simple principles it can be less complicated than unhealthy cooking, and can often even be thrown together in much the same time as it takes to peel the plastic off a ready meal and heat it up.

This chapter is designed to give you the simple strategies you need to make healthy cooking more effortless. With the help of our nutritional food consultant, Tina Deubert, we have brought you the building blocks for healthy stews, salads, curries and stir-fries, with basic methods to which you can add whatever ingredients you choose from the lists provided.

We haven't defined weights or mentioned calories and we have avoided counting or measuring food beyond rough volumes. This might make serial dieters feel uncertain at first, but over time it will bring you a healthy sense of liberation around food. Allowing yourself to connect with natural appetite, hunger and fullness signals is a crucial part of the De-Stress process and helps you feel the intuition you need to supply your body with the differing amounts it needs on different days.

Don't worry about getting 'out of control' around the food. As you are avoiding – where you can – trigger foods such as sugars, junk fats and refined carbohydrates, as well as identifying your stress cravings and false hunger, your body will begin to connect with the amounts it needs on different days during the 6-Week Plan.

If you're used to having lots of salt or sugary foods, it might take some time for your taste buds to acclimatize to the new tastes, but after about 3 weeks – perhaps less – you will see a shift towards enjoying more subtle and sophisticated flavourings.

Start experimenting and using cooking as one of your meditative activities, staying mindful and perhaps listening to relaxing music as you chop and prepare. You might have the odd slightly strange outcome, but that is the worst that can happen. If you're already a whizz in the kitchen, there's plenty to explore in the suggestions below to find the healthiest foods that suit your palate. Add your own twists, too, and make note of your favourite combinations to build a repertoire that encourages variety.

Lunch and Dinner Basics

All meals should supply:

- **Adequate protein** – meat, fish, eggs, nuts, some whole-fat dairy, some fully cooked legumes: 1/4 – 1/3 of a medium dinner plate or large bowl.

- **Plenty of the right complex carbohydrates** – plenty of vegetables (aim for 6–8 palm-sized portions daily) make up rest of your plate or bowl. If you're having starchy carbs like grains, beans, potatoes, sweet potatoes, parsnips, yams or cassava, stick to 1–2 a day. If beans are the protein part, just vegetables, no other starch, with added nuts/seeds should be your guide here.

- **Moderate 'good' fats** – in addition to the fat from meat, fish, eggs, nuts and whole-fat dairy, yoghurt and goat's cheese, coconut milk and oil, avocado, olive oil, olives and some vegetables provide the right kind of fats your body needs. Add an extra omega 3 oil supplement to address the deficit of this essential fatty acid in modern foods (see page 67).

Quantities and Sources

Ingredient	Amounts per person	Healthy Option
Vegetables	At least 1 handful of 3 or more kinds. Up to 3 cups at each meal	Organic where possible, see http://www.ewg.org/foodnews/list/ for foods to prioritize to lower your pesticide load
Meat	Palm-sized piece; prioritize quality over quantity and you may find you are satisfied with less.	Free-range, organic, grass-fed meat including game, liver and other organ meats where possible;[1] if wild or pasture-raised animal foods are hard to obtain, beef, lamb, butter and cheese; do not choose cured meats (bacon, ham) more than once or twice a week.[2,3]
Fish – oily	Palm-sized piece; 2–3 times a week max, to avoid toxic build-up	Sustainable, mercury-free wild fish and seafood; wild Alaskan salmon, mackerel, sardines, herring, anchovies, trout; avoid mercury-high tuna, swordfish and marlin.[4,5,6]
Fish – white and seafood	A palm-sized piece; good substitute for red meat	Sustainable and mercury-free sources, line-caught pollock, halibut, haddock; farmed clams, scallops, squid, prawns, shrimp
Eggs	1–2 a day	free-range, organic grass-fed chickens where possible
Dairy	Occasional small block feta or other cheese if tolerant. Tablespoon Greek live or whole milk live or 'bio' if tolerant	Prioritize organic where possible to avoid high levels of hormones and antibiotics[7] and for healthier fat profile.[8]
Beans/legumes/pulses	½ mug cooked volume	Organic, darker-coloured varieties such as black beans are higher in antioxidants.
Nuts	1 palmful maximum daily, in food or as a snack	Organic for best mineral levels; can soak or slow-cook otherwise oils oxidize when cooked
Seeds	Add liberally to salads	As for nuts
Tofu	Palm-sized piece up to twice a week max	See soy info page 40; choose good quality fermented types

Garlic	1–2 cloves depending on your tastes	Ideally organic fresh, cloves chopped or crushed. Can buy good quality 'quick' garlic paste in tubes, jars or frozen.
Turmeric, cinnamon, paprika, curry powder, cumin, coriander	About 1 tsp total – more if you like	Ground fine (organic where possible) unless you are a chef-extraordinaire and used to grinding yourself. Change regularly; if a spice has lost its smell, it needs replacing.
Fresh ginger	Up to ½in root, grated	Easy to buy fresh root in vegetable sections. Can also buy good quality 'quick' ginger paste in tubes or chopped in jars, which can be a better alternative to the much less pungent ground spice, but check for sugar or additives.
Dried herbs, bay leaves	About ½ tsp dried herbs/1 bay leaf	Buy in small quantities to replace often. Dried herbs are much less pungent than fresh, so you might use more.
Fresh herbs	A handful or more a day	Easiest to grow in pots in the kitchen or on the window sill; can be bought organically in good supermarkets to use liberally and freeze well.
Creamed coconut	Half to whole 200g block, grated or chopped fairly small	Buy organic blocks in health food shops or healthy section of supermarkets. You can chop off and add directly to cooking or make up milk by adding hot water; 200g creamed coconut makes about 600ml of thickish coconut milk.
Lemons/limes and their juice	Juice of 1 or 2, to taste	
Butter, coconut oil	For baking and cooking	Saturated fats are less damaging to body tissues when heated than polyunsaturated oils like sunflower. Buy organic where possible and unsalted butter so you can add a little high-quality salt if needed – see below. If you want a spreadable butter, look for one with least sunflower oil, so no 'low-fat' versions. Buy coconut oil from a health food shop where it can be guaranteed not to be deodorized or hydrogenated.

Olive oil	For cooking and salads	Unrefined, cold-pressed, virgin – buy quality for higher anti-inflammatory oleocanthal and oleic acid; to absorb fat-soluble nutrients from salads.
Sea or rock salt	Sprinkle for food	Can help tired adrenals when body low in sodium. Buy good quality, avoiding cheap table salts that are chemically processed and lack the extra minerals in some rock salts – iron gives Himalayan salt its pink colour.

DSD Tip

You'll notice we haven't recommended polyunsaturated oils like sun-flower oil. Some cold-pressed versions of these can be used for dress-ings, but the refined types bought in plastic bottles provide too many omega 6 oils, and toxins from the plastic easily leach into the oil. These should never be used for cooking as they are easily damaged by heat and produce harmful trans-fats.[9]

Stews, Casseroles, Curries

Can be eaten for lunch, dinner or even breakfast. You can leave them to slow-cook all day for your evening meal, put them in a flask for lunch or freeze them in portion-sized packs for another day. Most benefit from long, slow cooking – especially if you're including beans or grains like buckwheat groats or pearl barley. If you're short on time, put all in-gredients into a slow cooker (a fabulous, cheap De-Stress investment), cover with water and slow cook overnight to take in a thermos for work the next day, or leave to cook while you're at work so you've got a hot pot of food to come home to.

DSD Tip

Always cook with garlic and onions in abundance as do most tra-ditional cultures. They have shown to be anti-inflammatory, immune-modulating, antibacterial and to aid blood-sugar balance, circulation, detoxification and digestion.[10]

The Method

1. Choose your ingredients and the flavours you'd like.

2. Put some olive oil, butter or coconut oil in a pan.

3. Add onions, garlic and flavourings, and gently fry until they begin to soften.

4. Add vegetables and stir them around for a few minutes until they begin to soften.

5. Add the protein (this might be done earlier, depending on the amount of time it needs to cook).

6. Add water or homemade unsalted stock to cover all the ingredients twice over. Don't add salt at this stage if you are using soaked and uncooked beans or lentils (it makes the skins hard and difficult to digest). See below on the basic cooking method for beans. You can also add the woody herbs at this stage, like fresh thyme, rosemary and bay leaves.

7. Bring to the boil, simmer on a low heat and allow to cook for desired cooking time – this will depend on how long the protein part of your meal will take to cook. If you're not using a slow cooker, turn the heat to as low as it will go, cover, and remember to stir every so often to avoid sticking and burning; it will take 1–2 hours with meat and pulses, but if you're using pre-cooked pulses, tofu or fish it will be 30–45 minutes.

8. Before serving add some finely chopped spinach or steam some green vegetables, then add the final seasonings such as fresh chopped herbs, creamed coconut (grated or chopped up then stirred until dissolved), lemon or lime juice, sea/rock salt and pepper, tamarind paste (from Asian grocers) and/or yoghurt.

Flavouring

Choose from the following flavour 'families':

- Thai – chilli, coconut and lime with fresh ginger or green Thai curry paste

- Mediterranean – garlic, basil, oregano, rosemary, thyme, bay leaves and chilli
- Indian – ginger, garlic, cumin, coriander, turmeric and chilli or curry powder
- Moroccan – cinnamon, cumin, coriander, paprika, lemon (can be preserved)
- Herby – garlic, parsley, thyme, chives, bay leaves

    … or whatever combination you like.

Vegetables

Depending on season and availability, with a mixture of colours, for example:

- Celery
- Carrot
- Courgette
- Leek
- Savoy cabbage
- Squash/pumpkin
- Cauliflower
- Broccoli
- Mushrooms
- Fennel

Protein

- Meat
- Soaked beans (pre-cooked if you want a meal in a hurry, just soaked if you're leaving it on the slow cooker)
- Lentils

For 'softer' proteins, add them near the end of the cooking time:

- Cooked meats
- Cashew nuts
- Chestnuts
- Fish
- Cheese
- Tofu

Soups

Soups are similar to stews, but tend to be cooked more quickly for immediate use. You can make more than you need and take the rest to work the next day, or freeze in portions to defrost overnight or during the day for dinner. Use the same basic method mentioned above, adding enough water to cover the ingredients twice over. You will need to add more water if you're using lentils, beans or grains, as they will absorb most of it, so check after 20 minutes and add more water as necessary. Some soups will be better liquidized and others better served with 'bits' or 'chunkyness'. This will depend on your preference. Try both ways and decide for yourself. All will have onions, unless otherwise stated. Some contain protein such as meat or poultry; vegetarians can add pre-cooked pulses or sprinkle nuts and seeds on the top when serving. Split red lentils are a great protein to use with smooth soups.

Smooth Soups

These may provide less protein and make a less substantial meal, but can be eaten with sourdough rye or a large salad for a heartier meal to avoid sugar dips later on; add pumpkin seeds for protein:

- Split red lentils, carrots, spinach and coconut with turmeric, cumin, coriander (or curry powder)
- Celery, red pepper, carrot, basil

- Butternut or other orange squash/pumpkin, carrot and coriander

- Peas and mint with a dollop of Greek yoghurt; you can make this really quickly with frozen peas and bought mint sauce, or more slowly with soaked split green peas and fresh mint

- Carrot, orange and coriander with chilli

- Cauliflower, celery and fennel with dill seeds

- Watercress with Greek yoghurt

Chunky Soups

As substantial as you make them. Choices may include:

- Fish soup – tomatoes, chilli and basil with chunks of firm white fish and prawns, mussels and other shellfish, finished off with plenty of chopped fresh parsley.

- 'Thai' fish soup – as above, but no tomatoes. Use ginger, lime, chilli and/or green Thai curry paste, stock and water, add the fish, then coconut and fresh coriander.

- Chicken soup – add cooked chicken to a spring vegetable stock base and add a good sized dessertspoon of Thai green curry paste and the juice of half a lime. Garnish with fresh coriander and finely chopped spring onions for an oriental flavour.

- Spring vegetable – use diced brightly coloured vegetables like carrot, peppers, celery, courgette and some greens, in a clear bouillon, finished with parsley. Add black beans or cooked chicken for protein.

- Root vegetable – carrot, parsnip, swede, turnip, with curry flavours and coconut with red lentils, black, mung or aduki beans; add lots of fresh chopped coriander at the end.

Flavourful Additions

- Add a good dollop of tahini when blending soups – it adds calcium and zinc, and makes the soup creamy (without dairy), thickening it slightly.

- Creamed coconut, which comes in a block. Shave slivers off and add near the end, stirring until dissolved and evenly distributed.
- Lemon, lime, orange or grapefruit juice add 'zing'.
- Natural Greek yoghurt added at the end.
- Lightly dry-roasted seed mix.
- Thai green curry paste to make any dull soup delicious.
- Herbs – fresh, chopped parsley, coriander and mint as garnish add a lovely fresh flavour and even more goodness.
- Finely chopped spinach added at the end to brighten up the soup, giving it a healthy green glow.

Salads

A salad can be any kind of raw and sometimes cooked vegetable, arranged together to form an attractive, colourful meal. Go for lots of colour using at least four types of vegetables, add flavoursome bits, some protein and a delicious dressing, and you have a satisfying meal rather than a boring side dish. Use an attractive pasta bowl or soup plate to hold your salad, and build it up in layers, such as those listed here, or just throw together what you fancy.

Layer 1

A handful of mixed green leaves, spread out to cover the bottom of the bowl:

- Lettuce, especially the darker varieties like romaine/cos
- Watercress
- Rocket
- Baby spinach leaves (or larger leaves 'cooked'*)
- Baby beetroot leaves (ditto)
- Herb leaf salad
- Mustard leaves

*With spinach or beet leaves there is the option to put them roughly chopped in a colander in the sink, then pour a kettle-full of boiling water over them to soften them up. Transfer to a bowl or jug and mix in some salad dressing, then leave to cool slightly before using in your salad.

Layer 2

Some of the following:

- Avocado

- Onion or spring onion, finely chopped

- Celery

- Fennel – raw slices

- Steamed asparagus

- Grilled artichokes (from deli counter)

- Cucumber

- Olives

- Roasted vegetables – warm or cold, anything that keeps its shape like fennel, celery, red pepper, cherry tomatoes, courgette, whole garlic cloves, small onions, sweet potatoes roasted with some olive oil and optional rosemary

- Handful of any roughly chopped fresh herb leaf

Layer 3

Optional raw root vegetables, grated:

- Carrot

- Beetroot

- Celeriac

- Courgette

Layer 4

Protein:

- Fish, meat or seafood – cold cuts, roasted meat or fish with olive oil and garlic, pan-fried slivers of liver, steak, duck, lamb, chicken or fish, still warm (Charlotte's quick favourite: baked salmon fillet or chicken breast slathered in pesto)

- Cooked beans/pulses/lentils

- Handful of raw nuts or seeds like sunflower, pumpkin and sesame

- Hardboiled egg

- Goat's or sheep's cheese, like feta or halloumi

Dressings and Tasty Additions

- The easiest and quickest dressing is 1–2 tbsp extra-virgin olive oil and a smaller splash of cider vinegar, balsamic vinegar or lemon juice, straight onto the salad.

- Olive oil, cider or wine vinegar, Dijon or wholegrain mustard and a tiny bit of honey, mixed together in a jar.

- Tahini, equal quantity of water, crushed garlic, juice of half a lemon (or more to taste) and a splash of soy sauce. Add a little bit of chilli too, if you like.

- A good-sized dollop of hummus (Note: this qualifies as a bean portion, so not if you're having a grain as well).

- Healthy sprinkles: Lightly toasted or raw seeds or nuts, crispy onions, pickled or black garlic, capers, soaked seaweed, anchovies, fennel or cumin seeds, baba ganoush, sprinkle of goat's cheese, a little rock or sea salt.

With the dressing applied, a salad will last in the fridge for two consecutive meals, so you could have it for lunch, dinner or even breakfast, or dinner and then the following day's lunch.

Stir-fries

Forget the idea of cooking at very high temperatures – lower temperatures give you time to stir and check with less chance of burning, and if you have a lid for your wok you can steam-fry (add water to the wok), giving you time to prepare other parts of the meal. Have a great big bowl, with more vegetables. You can miss out on the grain part if you are on the first 3 weeks of your De-Stress Success plan, or if you have decided to avoid them altogether. Alternatively, have a half a mug of grains and 2–3 cups of the vegetables as a good balance.

Always begin by sautéing onions. Then add:

Group 1 Vegetables
Cut into equal sized batons/sticks:
- Carrots
- Celery
- Peppers
- Mushrooms
- Leeks
- Kohlrabi

Group 2 Vegetables
Shredded:
- Broccoli
- Kale
- Cabbage
- Asparagus
- Bok choi/pak choi
- Spring greens
- Spinach
- Chard
- Brussels sprouts

Protein

- Raw or cooked meat
- Prawns
- White firm fish
- Cashew nuts
- Roasted almonds
- Tofu – cook this separately*

*To cook the tofu, cut into cubes and fry in a shallow layer of coconut oil, until lightly brown on all sides. Then tip into a bowl containing a mixture of soy sauce, finely grated ginger, crushed garlic and chilli. Stir it around, then return to the pan and stir and fry until dry and sticky. Put aside to add at the end.

You can give the meat and fish the same kind of treatment, and experiment with the flavourings. It works particularly well with leftover lamb or duck.

Method

1. Melt 1–2 tablespoons coconut oil in a wok, deep frying pan or a large saucepan.

2. Add one medium onion per person, stir and fry for 2 or 3 minutes.

3. Add crushed garlic – as much as you like, and grated fresh ginger – at least 1 dessertspoon.

4. Add Group 1 vegetables and stir-fry for a couple of minutes. Put the lid on if you have one, otherwise continue stirring and frying for about 5 minutes until they are beginning to soften.

5. Finely sliced raw meat can go in at this stage – stir and fry until nearly cooked.

6. Add the green vegetables along with softer proteins like fish, prawns and cooked meats; add a little water to steam with the lid on.

7. Continue to stir and fry for a few minutes until the greens just begin to wilt and the meat or fish is cooked.

8. Add the tofu, cashew nuts or the separately cooked meat at this stage and sprinkle with fresh chopped coriander.

Grains and Beans

Cooking to Reduce Phytic Acid and Lectins

Soak overnight, change the water in the morning and leave to soak again during the day. Change the water again and then cook for 1–2 hours depending on the type and age of bean. If you do large batches you can freeze portion-sized bags once they've cooled, and you'll have a ready supply to use in salads or cooking, without the toxic metals present in tins. You don't have to defrost them before use if cooking.

Add Vegetables

Cooking grains and beans with vegetables has shown to help reduce their phytic acid content, especially when slow-cooked to break it down further.[11,12] Grains and beans are traditionally cooked with garlic and onion to make iron and zinc more available; other members of this allium family – shallots, spring onions, leeks, scallions and chives – will also work, as well as providing insulin-regulating, circulation-supporting sulphur compounds.

Team Them Well

Eat grains and beans with foods rich in vitamin A and carotenoids (fat-soluble nutrients) found in meat, butter and deep-coloured vegetables, especially orange roots and dark green leaves.[13]

Try Sprouting

This has been shown to decrease phytic acid but increase levels of toxic lectins to protect young plants as they grow.[14] Traditional cultures sprout their grains and beans but then always cook them, so sprout then add to stews. Sprouting has shown to increase 'bioaccessibility' or availability of iron.[15]

Use Acidifiers

These are flavourings added to cooking that also break down anti-nutrients. They include amchur (or amchoor – mango powder – from Asian grocers), lime powder, tamarind, fruit, dried fruit, fruit juice – all of which can be added to soaking or cooking – and yoghurt, for a lactic acid pre-soak.[16]

If You Are Vegan

You need to take more care to soak beans and grains for at least 24 hours (changing the water at least once or twice) before cooking with an acidifier and eating alongside foods high in vitamin C (e. g. different coloured vegetables in a side salad) to help iron absorption. These can be pre-cooked and frozen in portions. Heat-cooking grains and beans has been shown to increase iron bioavailability but to decrease that of zinc[17] – commonly low in vegans.

Best Grain Choices

Depending on your tastes and energy needs, you may wish to add a small portion of grains to your breakfast or lunch. Try and minimize wheat to reduce the gluten in your diet, and vary the types of grains you choose from the list below so that you don't subject your immune system to the same lectins over and again.[18] The following are all gluten-free:

- **Quinoa and wild rice** – the most alkalizing grains

- **Basmati brown rice** – best for blood sugar but extremely high in phytic acid, so limit to 2–3 times a week

- **Millet and buckwheat** – cause the fewest immune reactions

- **Buckwheat groats** – great in stews; not related to wheat

- **Sweet potatoes** – less starchy than potatoes

- **New potatoes** – skins intact, the best potato choice; have baked potatoes as an occasional lunch treat only

Chapter 7

TAKING THE STRESS
OUT OF LUNCH

If you're wondering why so many of us feel exhausted at our desks by 4 o'clock in the afternoon, here's food for thought: seven out of ten office workers don't leave their desks at lunchtime, and a staggering seven million skip lunch breaks altogether. Even for those of us who do take time out, our lunch breaks have shrunk to an all-time low and now last around 36 minutes.[1] Instead of a quick refuelling on the run (if we're lucky), a healthy, well-thought out – but not necessarily high-maintenance – lunch is an essential component of the De-Stress Diet.

During the course of the average high-pressure day, demands are put on our bodies in terms of functioning, maintenance and recovery. That means the essential nutrients we need to cope with the mental stress we're under – B vitamins, vitamin C, magnesium and zinc, to name a few – are quickly used up by the body's stress response. Unless we choose meals that replenish these nutrients we can soon be running on empty and find ourselves turning to stimulants such as coffee, chocolate and crisps to keep us going instead. A decent lunch is a great chance to refuel intelligently, 'top up' your daily De-Stress routine and keep your mind fresh and able to cope with the day's demands. It can also provide slow-feed energy and nutrients from good-quality proteins and vegetables to help regulate the highs and lows of energy that can lead to cravings and symptoms of stress later in the day.

Lunchtime Pick-me-ups

Get Some Light

A10-minute walk to a nearby park or café can ensure you get a hit of vitamin D, especially in the winter when you may not see any daylight during the morning or evening hours. If it's a dull day, try and be outside at lunchtime for half an hour or more, finding oxygenating greenery if you can. If the sun is out, 10 minutes will be enough to optimize vitamin D production – especially if you're not wearing sunscreen.

Make It a Meal

The average person spends about £2.50 on lunch each day, and we're not about to start asking you to start fine dining and splashing out more cash.[2] With just a little planning you can make a meal out of lunch for £2.50 a day or less. We urge you to make your own where you can; the previous chapter has easy and low-maintenance advice on how. Even if you only commit to doing this a few days a week, it will help promote the feeling that you are looking after yourself and making the healthiest choices you can. Plus, because you will be cooking more easy De-Stress dinners at home, you will have healthy leftovers to bring into work for lunch the next day. The money you save can be spent on better-quality shop-bought lunches on those days when you don't bring your own.

Pack in the Protein

Make about 30 per cent of your lunch protein (this is about a quarter of your plate) in the form of lean meat, eggs, fish (smoked or fresh), nuts, seeds, pulses or beans – or a mix of these. Protein takes longer to digest and will keep you well-fuelled and feeling fuller for longer.

If you can't afford or find organic varieties of meat, read the labels to ensure you're buying wild or free-range options to which no sugars, salts, processed fats or preservatives such as sodium or potassium nitrate have been added. Omelets or frittatas made with plenty of vegetables (and a little feta cheese) and eaten with a huge salad on the side make for a great protein-rich lunch and you can slice off portions from the fridge for a few meals.

Bulk Up on Vegetables

Vegetables and salad should make up the bulk of your lunch, especially green leafy vegetables where you can. Super salads with plenty of avocado, fresh herb leaves, greens such as watercress, rocket or chicory and lots of brightly coloured vegetables such as grated beetroots, carrots and courgettes, sliced tomatoes, cucumbers, celery and peppers should accompany your protein choice at least four times a week.

As outlined in the previous chapter, soups are a great way of getting your vegetable nutrients and naturally hydrate. You can prepare them beforehand and freeze in containers to bring into work in a large thermos or to warm up in the microwave at lunchtime.

When You Have to Go Store-Bought

If you have little time and need to go for store-bought options, make the healthiest choice you can. We have some general advice to make this easier for you, and if you log on to de-stressyourlife.com you will find specific approved options from M&S, Sainsbury's, Pret, EAT and Tesco within our 6-week Plan Support emails. (See, we're always thinking of you.)

Lab Chat: Vinegar and GI

A study from Arizona State University found that adding vinegar to food lowers its Glycaemic Index (GI), so helps to control insulin levels and keep you full longer.[3] Lemon juice also has the same effect and both help digestion by raising acidity in the stomach. Stress-related low stomach acid also causes indigestion after meals, when undigested food mixed with stomach acid rises back into the oesophagus. Use with caution if you have a stomach ulcer, though.

Lunchtime Dos and Don'ts

Do

- Use lunch to increase your vegetable intake. Having vegetables only at dinner won't provide enough of the fibre, vitamins and minerals a stressed body needs.

- Experiment during your 6-Week Plan with grains or beans at lunch. One serving is about half a cup, and always have grains or beans, not both. Some people find that grains actually increase their appetite and make them sleepy, so they choose only protein and vegetables at lunch. Use the Troubleshooters on page 119 and the De-Stress Progress Charts on pages 223–31 to help you.

- If you're buying out, look for shops that sell alternatives to wheat bread such as rye or wholegrain (if you really want a sandwich) and avoid malted breads, as the brown colour comes from the addition of *maltose*, a form of sugar. Even some train station chains now sell sourdough wheat, which is a better alternative. Flat breads can contain fewer additives, and the odd wrap, although high in refined carbohydrates, may be tolerated better by those with digestive issues.

Don't

- Have a sandwich every day. If you do eat bread, have several days off gluten-containing wheat (or rye) each week by choosing a super soup or salad as an alternative.

- Choose refined carbohydrates. White bread, pastries and pies release energy too quickly and provide 'empty' calories that quickly turn to fat. Wouldn't dream of eating cake for lunch? Having such refined carbohydrates is, in nutritional terms, very similar.

Cheap and Healthy Options

Freezer Batch

See Chapter 6 for easy stew or curry ideas to make in bulk on a Sunday night, leaving to cool and creating separate portions in airtight containers to freeze. If you take one to work, heat up in the microwave or defrost overnight to heat in the morning and take in a thermos flask.

At-work Lunch Store Cupboard

If you have a fridge and a small storage and preparation space at work, try keeping a capsule store cupboard and topping it up regularly. For tasty and inexpensive lunches, the idea is to have the makings of a great lunch ready and waiting so that, come lunchtime, all you need do is assemble them into what you feel like. Mix and match ingredients to make a different lunch each day.

Buy Monthly

- Extra-virgin olive oil

- Balsamic or apple cider vinegar, or bottled lemon juice

- Salmon, sardines and mackerel, lentils, chickpeas, cannellini and broad beans

- Bags of sunflower and pumpkin seeds

Buy Weekly

- 2–3 lemons for dressing

- small tub of hummus, Greek yoghurt and/or full-fat cottage cheese with chives

- 1 bunch romaine, iceberg or cos lettuce

- 1 bag watercress or rocket

- 1 punnet baby tomatoes

- 2 avocados

- container of fresh grated beetroot or ready-cooked without vinegar

- Other vegetables available that can be eaten raw – radishes, red onion, cucumber, fennel, mangetout etc.

- pre-cooked brown rice (optional, only if you're eating grains) will keep in fridge for a few days

- fresh, preferably organic roasted chicken, turkey breast or Parma ham (check it's not preserved with nitrates)

How You Have Lunch

Nourishing yourself isn't only about what you eat, but how you eat it. Here's the ideal De-Stress lunch routine, with options depending on the situation and how much time you have.

Your Stress-free Lunchtime

- About four or five hours after breakfast or when you begin to feel hungry, stop, leave your desk and go and prepare or buy your lunch. Take 10 deep breaths before leaving your desk to help punctuate the end of the morning and calm any leftover stress response that could hinder your digestion.

- Having your own brought-in lunch in a park with a friend ticks many De-Stress boxes. If you can't manage this, a café or restaurant is better than your desk. If the weather is awful, use a staff room or any location you can for lunch – other than your desk. Look for somewhere that gives you a chance to socialize with colleagues (you like), as this provides a social rest quick fix.

Those Stressy Habits Resolved

- Try and resist the urge to nip to the nearest unhealthy take-away and instead stroll somewhere where you know there is better choice. Try and avoid any ready meals.

- Only go for a walk if you have allowed 15 minutes to digest. It is better to rest and promote recharging, especially if you have digestive issues.

- Plan a walk for an afternoon break, even 5 minutes round your building or the block.

- If you like your coffee, have it after lunch. This will help slow down the rate at which coffee releases adrenaline into your system and prevent you feeling stress later in the afternoon. Swap a milky latte for a one-shot Americano with a little hot milk.

Making the Transition Work for You

Here are some ways to gradually transform your current lunch into a healthier, more De-Stressing one:

Stressy lunch	Finding Your Balance	De-Stress Success
Nothing – I have a deadline!	Take 10 deep breaths and then at least have a small version of a lunch. If you tend to skip lunch when you have a deadline, a few carrot sticks and six Brazil nuts will help balance your blood-sugar until the stressful event has passed.	Try to get into the habit of eating a healthy lunch even on days when you have a deadline. Ask yourself, 'How will skipping lunch make me feel later?' Remember that skipping lunch now may affect your work performance at the very time you need maximum brain power, and set you off on a stress cycle.
Ready meal	See the instructions above for making a salad as quickly as heating a ready meal. Alternatively, try our freezer batch lunch options in the last chapter. If this is still too high-maintenance, a bought-in soup is a good alternative.	Look for high-protein soups such as pea and ham, goulash and hearty lentils to help keep you going. Ensure your portion is big enough to satisfy you – a large bowl! If you have to have a ready meal, check labels for ingredients you simply don't recognize as food and avoid them. Indian and spicy dishes often have fewer preservatives as the spices themselves preserve food well.

A bought-in salad that never satisfies me	When you're choosing a store-bought salad, ensure it is high enough in protein and good fat to satisfy you for the rest of the afternoon.	Look for a salad that contains protein equivalent to the palm of your hand, and also comes with good fats in the form of any one or two of the following: avocado, olives, rapeseed, olive or sesame oil, a few mixed nuts or seeds. Check your dressing label for sugar content – a ready-made salad dressing labelled 'low-fat' may be high in sugar. The 'gloopy' pasta or potato 'salad' choice is never the good option.
Client lunches with good wine on offer	You will probably be expected to have a thimbleful of wine so if you feel that saying no isn't an option, have a couple of glasses of water before you leave so you don't arrive thirsty and drink wine to get hydrated (doesn't work). Add some sparkling mineral water or a few ice cubes to your wine to stop the alcohol hitting your system too quickly. Remember, though, it's now completely acceptable not to drink at lunchtime (or any other time, for that matter!) and peer group pressure really is unacceptable.	To avoid this becoming a starchy carb and poor-quality fat fest, make sure you choose a dish with adequate protein such as egg, salmon, chicken, seafood or ham and have the sauce on the side, with an extra side serving of vegetables. If having alcohol, the protein and veg will help your liver handle it. Try and swap some client lunches for breakfast, morning or afternoon tea in which you will be under less of an obligation to eat and drink whatever is on offer.

Troubleshooting: Lunch

Making time for lunch helps the way you feel for the rest of the day. Here are some ideas for times when life gets in the way of your best De-Stress lunch intentions:

PROBLEM: *You feel guilty because no one else is having lunch.*

SOLUTION: Claim this time as your own necessary recovery space because it makes you more productive. Leaving lunch too late and letting yourself get too hungry before lunch can lead to a plummet in your blood-sugar and a need to eat anything you can get your hands on. This can also leave you irritable and far more inclined to eat a larger amount than you need. Try to leave no more than five hours between breakfast and lunch. If you really do need a snack to fill the blood-sugar gap before lunch, choose the healthiest options on pages 142–43.

PROBLEM: *You get bloated after lunch whatever you eat.*

SOLUTION: Pre-lunch, take 10 long, slow breaths. When we are stressed our digestion suffers, which can leave us bloated or gassy after eating. Getting into this habit will relax your body and minimize any stress response. You might have a hidden wheat or gluten intolerance (see page 32 and <u>de-stressyourlife.com</u> for suggestions on getting tested). Try and avoid wheat-containing sandwiches, pizza, noodles, pastas and quiches. Add dried spices such as anise, fennel and ginger to your lunch to aid digestion and help combat bloating or flatulence. Choose potassium-rich vegetables such as cucumbers, parsley and asparagus, as these have a diuretic effect that can help keep your tummy flat. Add fresh herbs to food to calm and soothe digestion.

PROBLEM: *You go to the gym at lunchtime.*

SOLUTION: Try and take a slightly earlier lunch break for your workout so you can still eat before blood-sugar levels dip. If you normally work out at 1 p.m. and then eat, by the time the workout is over low blood-sugar could make you eat more than you need, and/or crave sugary foods. Have a small, easily digestible snack pre-exercise to ensure good fuel to muscles, like a piece of fruit

15 minutes before. Refuel immediately afterwards and prioritize protein, especially if you are doing the De-Stress 25-minute resistance workout, after which your muscles will need refuelling. Great sources of post-workout protein include smoked salmon, eggs, fish, prawns, goat's cheese; if you are a vegan, a portion of nuts or beans.

. . . .

PROBLEM: *You get so hungry you're tempted to order the most unhealthy thing on the menu.*

SOLUTION: Don't mistake hearty for unhealthy. You might consider it unhealthy but a hot meal of delicious grilled or roasted fish, chicken or lean lamb with multi-coloured vegetables is a healthier option than some restaurant salads and will provide the amino acids and energy that your brain and body need to function through the day. It will also make it less likely that you overeat at dinner.

. . . .

PROBLEM: *You don't feel satisfied without something sweet after lunch.*

SOLUTION: Be assured that this tendency is a body and mind conditioning that can change. Reduce sugars elsewhere in your diet and follow the recommendations on page 147 to move away from sugar. Have a herbal tea with licorice and/or cinnamon to help regulate insulin and tell your brain you've received something sweet. A portion of berries is the best sweet choice. The supplements recommended in the 6-Week Plan help to curb sweet cravings. Ensure your multivitamin contains 400mcg chromium, consider an extra supplement or one within a dedicated 'glucose tolerance' formulation containing chromium.

Help by Stress Suit		
	You may find that you...	**Best single change you could make**
Stressed and Wired	are far too busy to stop for lunch	Even adding 5–10 minutes to your break can make a difference. If you're really pushed, have a hearty soup that is easier to digest.
Stressed and Tired	feel an energy slump after lunch	See the caffeine section on page 152. Try licorice tea for natural energy production.
Stressed and Cold	feel tired from the morning's activities	Make sure you get some cold or fresh air, particularly if your office is stuffy. Even if you hate the idea, it will soon invigorate you.
Stressed and Bloated	bloat or feel discomfort after eating lunch	Follow your lunch with dandelion, mint, fennel or nettle tea – all great bloating-relievers.
Stressed and Sore	can feel stress-related inflammatory symptoms rising after lunch	Keep a food diary to monitor which types of lunch affect you. Take an extra vitamin C with lunch when needed as a natural anti-histamine; you may need more when stressed.
Stressed and Demotivated	feel you might need to console yourself with 'bad' foods	Phone a trusted friend who makes you laugh instead, or pick a breathing exercise that makes you feel centred.
Stressed and Hormonal	just want sweet foods before and around the time of your period	If you need to succumb, be very clear about choosing quality treats and then enjoy only after a healthy lunch.

Chapter 8

DE-STRESSING DINNER

Just as what you do and eat in the morning sets the tone for how you will feel and function throughout the day, so your evening routine sets the tone for the next morning. Yet we often fight our natural impulse towards a relaxing, sleep-inducing evening, believing we might be missing out if we're not having an extremely exciting time. In the modern world this often means drinking alcohol if out with friends or tech-overload if staying in. Looking at how these activities affect our sleep can help us find a balance between enjoyment, health and weight loss.

The essence of the De-Stress Diet is approaching daytime in such a way that we can sail into the evening and feel ready for sleep when it comes. We are not suggesting you become a monastic hermit, eschewing any excitement in the evening, but you can stay mindful of how much you might need to recover from the stress assault of the day and how enjoyable this can be. Evening is the time when cortisol levels are lowering to reduce stimulation and prepare the body for rest. Stress taken into the evening can not only keep you awake, it can increase the likelihood of your body laying down fat.[1] Evening relaxation helps keep your appetite appropriate for the low level of activity that your body expects at night, and helps your digestion at a time when it is slowing down.

Those hours when you are unconscious are some of the most important in your life.[2] In order for you to function fully while awake, your body relies on the immune-modulation, detoxification, tissue- and muscle-healing and mental-sorting processes that occur during this time.[3] If you don't respect this, chances are you will experience fatigue, irritability, poor concentration and poor recovery from stress, injury and skin complaints.

Your brain is only around 3 per cent of your body weight but it uses around a quarter of your energy, requiring lots of recovery time.

Tired, But Not Sleepy

Chronic tiredness at night is common, and often about physical difficulties dealing with stress. After days of commuting, looking after children, working 8–18 hours with no lunch-break and evenings spent texting or surfing the net, it's understandable to feel exhausted at the end of the day. Our body clocks – that is, the 24-hour daily metabolic rhythms set into our biochemistry – have been set from when we lived in caves.[4] They follow the light–dark cycles of the sun, but continue even when we don't see daylight.[5] This means ideally waking on sunrise and going to bed at sunset, obviously not something your average 21st-century dweller is doing. Simply putting lights on when it is dark outside, watching TV and surfing the net disrupt this system, which is naturally designed to shut you down for rest and recovery.[6] Our ancestors would have wound down by socializing with the tribe, chatting, eating, dancing and having sex – all De-Stress evening activities we highly recommend.

DSD Tip

A nap of 15–30 minutes mid-afternoon can help prevent us relying on stress hormones or stimulants when getting enough sleep eludes us. Any longer and moving into deeper sleep cycles can result in grogginess rather than rejuvenation.[7]

Sleep-supporters

Consider trying the following for at least half of your week, or have a monthly 'holiday at home' with the activities below each night for a week. This is great for stressful times when your sleep has become affected and you have slipped into those over-stimulating evening habits.

- Evaluate where your social life might be draining rather than recharging you. Does one night out make you feel connected and happy, whereas two in a row leave you having difficulty falling asleep and prone to craving refined carbs the next day?

- See the alcohol section on pages 156–59 to learn about going out without regrets.

- Communicate only with people who make you feel comforted and safe, not whipping up difficult emotional issues at a time when you need your brain to relax. This includes phone conversations, well-chosen social media and real physical interaction.

- Avoid all stimulants past 4 p.m. – caffeine, alcohol, sugar and excessive TV or computer use once you're home from work.

- Anything you do towards the end of the day should be moving you towards a calm 'alpha' brain state: baths, reading non-thrilling books, listening to soothing music, a calm yoga practice or meditation will ensure quality rest.

- Don't fight it if you're tired: go to bed early and allow yourself to catch up on sleep.

- Aim to have as consistent as possible a bed-time and wake-time, to let your body feel safe in its rhythm. Aim to be in bed by 11 p.m. as often as possible; the hours before midnight can be more restorative than those after.

- Sleep in a chilly and fully dark room (like our ancestors' caves). Too much heat or light can halt the production of melatonin.

- Switch off as many electrical devices in your bedroom as you can. Electro-Magnetic Fields (EMFs) from cordless phone, wireless and mobile-charging hubs can disrupt your sleep quality.

Evening Exercise

For many, the evening is the only time they can find to exercise, but leave it too late and the nervous system excitation this can cause can affect sleep neurotransmitters. Our best cardiovascular efficiency and muscle strength is around 5 p.m.,[14] so straight after work is a great time to exercise and best for the heart. Exercising outside helps to keep you connected to the natural world in terms of daylight and temperature, whereas more bright lights might tell your body artificially that it is another time of day entirely. If evening is your chosen time, end with something that actively calms your nervous system. See the yoga sequence and breathing exercise in Chapter 11. Even just one restorative posture or 10 minutes of focused breathing can calm you down for a restful night's sleep.

Evening Food

Living in the 21st century means we're far removed from the 5 p.m. 'tea time' that was a staple a generation or two ago. Now, many of us – the authors included – may not get home until 8 p.m., at which point the last thing we feel like doing is spending hours cooking our evening meals. This can leave us at the mercy of heat-and-eat ready meals and eating later than our bodies want to digest. The De-Stress Diet will minimize the effects of this by prioritizing breakfast and lunch as larger meals, to help accommodate your energy and nutrient needs throughout the day so you don't get home as famished, and feel better-equipped to make healthier choices in the evening.

After the first 3 weeks of your De-Stress Diet, your body should begin to get used to being fed better during the day. Without a string of blood-sugar highs and lows, you may become less inclined to overeat at night and your body has a chance to regenerate and rebuild itself during sleep rather than working overtime to digest an oversized evening meal.

You may go through a few days when your evening meal doesn't seem filling enough, but this will help to wake up morning hunger so you want a more satisfying breakfast, crucial if you've been skipping it. This chapter will show you how to make the right choices to help your brain generate its own essential evening neurotransmitters (nervous system messengers), such as melatonin and serotonin, which it needs for sound sleep and mood stabilization, especially during times of chronic stress.

Sleep Nutrient: Magnesium[8]		
What	**Sources**	**Need to Know**
Normal supplementation range: 300–700mg	In balance with calcium: green leafy vegetables, nuts, seeds, fish, carrots, sweet potato, avocado, cauliflower, tahini, parsley; occasional soy, whole grains, lentils	Modern man can tend to get more calcium and less magnesium than Stone Age from more dairy and fewer green leaves. As these two 'calming minerals' work together (balance anywhere between 2:1 and 1:1 is much discussed), many people benefit from extra magnesium to be able to use both.
Best forms as citrate or amino acid chelate		
Glycine and taurine forms can help produce sleep neurotransmitters in the evening.		
Only take calcium or bone-health supplements with magnesium included.		Magnesium deficiency can show up as any symptom relating to nervous system agitation: anxiety, insomnia, headaches, muscle cramps, PMS, depression, fatigue, fibromyalgia, panic attacks, IBS, blood-sugar issues.[9,10,11,12,13]
Can take 300–400mg evenings to promote sleep, and extra in the morning to help prevent anxiety where needed.		

Optimizing serotonin and other inhibitory or calming neurotransmitters also helps levels of GABA, the calming chemical that helps us switch off[15] and supports immunity.[16] Clearly we all want a dose of this to go to sleep, but the ability to produce GABA reaches into the daytime, too, low levels being associated with anxiety, panic attacks and mental health issues as well as insomnia.

DSD Tip

Vitamin B$_6$ is the only B vitamin recommended at night. Others can stimulate, but B$_6$ is needed to produce GABA[17] and serotonin and works with magnesium. A supplement up to 50mg can be taken with dinner.

Glutamine-rich De-Stress foods, which help produce GABA:

*   bananas
*   broccoli
*   citrus fruits
*   halibut
*   lentils
*   nuts
*   organ meats

Tryptophan-rich De-Stress foods, which help produce serotonin:

*   almonds
*   avocados
*   bananas
*   beetroot
*   chicken
*   cottage cheese
*   duck
*   figs
*   mackerel
*   pheasant
*   salmon
*   sunflower seeds
*   tofu
*   turkey

Dinner Guidelines

Make Dinner Your Smallest Meal of the Day

Try and eat a little less in the evenings and go to bed a little hungry so that you have an appetite for breakfast the next morning. It takes around 10 minutes for your stomach to signal fullness to the brain, so give that a chance to happen. Try and eat between 6.30 and 8 p.m. if you can.

Eat Protein and Vegetables

Having adequate protein in the evenings is essential, as protein contains amino acids that your body can only get from food and that it needs for the rebuilding processes that it will perform at night. For simple evening meal portion control, make a quarter of your plate protein and the other three-quarters vegetables.

No Starchy Carbs

If you choose to include grains, beans and potatoes in your diet, have them at breakfast or lunch. If you're eating out, avoid the pasta, potatoes and bread basket and have an extra side order of vegetables instead.

Avoid Puddings and Sweets

Save these for a very occasional treat. Eating sugar, crisps and chocolate in the evenings promotes an insulin surge and stimulates a blood-sugar spike before bed. This can interfere with sleep and promote weight gain.

Have a Bedtime Snack

If you tend to wake in the wee hours, see below for what you can do at dinner to help prevent this. A bedtime snack can help keep your blood-sugar stable – especially when you are stressed and using up your nutrients more quickly. It can also help support the production of serotonin. In chapter 9 you will find more suggestions for bedtime snacks that can help promote a good night's sleep.

Eat for Sleep

This still counts when you're out for dinner. No, you don't want to fall asleep in your soup, but you are still preparing for bed on a biochemical level, and what you eat in the evening will always have a direct impact on the way you sleep.

Those susceptible to insomnia can be sensitive to the excitory amino acid tyramine, and so should try to avoid eating any of these foods in the evening:[18]

• strong cheese

• chocolate

- aged or fermented foods like sauerkraut, soy sauce, tofu, miso, yeast extracts

- bacon, sausage, smoked meats, salami

- pickled and salted fish

- beer, ale and wine

- broad beans

DSD Tip

Taste is most acute in the evening, so bland meals might leave you wanting more.[19] See the flavouring guidelines on page 101.

Smart Dining

If you're out to dinner, opt for a light salad starter and avoid dessert. The best starters 'whet the appetite' and stimulate digestive juices so you can better assimilate the nutrients in your main course. These are usually bitter or sour foods that stimulate the pancreas to produce bile, which helps you digest the meal to come. Great choices of bile-promoting bitter and sour foods include grapefruit, olives, watercress, artichoke, chicory, parsley and radicchio. Avoid creamy dressings and instead liven up your meat, fish, pulses and vegetables with olive oil, fresh lemon juice, herbs such as parsley, unsalted butter, garlic, spices, mustard, vinegar and freshly made dressings.

Healthy Take-away and Dining Out Options

Italian

Avoid large bowls of pasta – choose a salad which includes egg, fresh anchovies, chicken, asparagus, avocado or rocket.

If you want pasta ask for a small side portion.

Avoid the bread basket or garlic bread.

Avoid pizza, but if this is one of your treats, have a small thin-crust one, avoid pepperoni and other fatty toppings, choose good quality where you can and have a little mozzarella rather than oceans of cheddar and load up the vegetables instead. Alternatively, share a pizza and a salad with a friend.

Indian

Choose chicken tandoori or tikka without a sauce and have with a vegetable side dish.

Try dahl (lentil curry) instead of rice or naan bread.

If you can, prepare a small portion of wild or brown Basmati rice at home to accompany, rather than the usual white rice, or just have half your usual amount, steamed not fried.

Ask for dishes with coconut instead of cream; avoid masalas and kormas.

If having a curry, ask for vegetables to be added.

Avoid deep-fried accompaniments like bhajis, poppadoms or pakoras.

Thai

Avoid large bowls of noodles or white rice. See the rice suggestions for Indian food.

Choose a healthy green or red curry.

Choose grilled fish with a vegetable accompaniment.

Have a vegetable side dish – something simple with ginger and/or lime can be healthy and clean tasting.

Avoid deep-fried accompaniments like crab cakes or battered prawns.

How You Have Dinner

Here's the ideal De-Stress dinner routine, with options depending on the amount of time you have to devote to it.

Your Stress-free Dinnertime

- Come home and prepare dinner for yourself and/or family. If you feel stressed and hungry when you get home, be mindful of what you're doing (even if it's chopping vegetables), how you're feeling and tune into your breathing, is it rushed? Shallow? Accept how you're feeling and observe your breath slowing down. If you feel you need to eat something, have six almonds or half an avocado with some lemon juice and black pepper. The fat in these foods will satisfy you without ruining your appetite.

- Have some coconut water or a 'mocktail' such as a Virgin Mary with plenty of black pepper and celery. These drinks will help re-hydrate your body instead of dehydrate it (like wine).

- Do a simple mindfulness exercise (see page 198) as you prepare dinner.

- Play some classical music when you get home – if you have some Bach or Brahms, great, but anything soothing is fine. This will stimulate your parasympathetic nervous system and help you and the family relax into your evening.

- Sit at the table for dinner. Set the table in an appealing way, with a simple bunch of flowers or low candle. This will help make dinner an event and get the family talking across the table.

- Truly relax and chew while you eat to aid full digestion and helping your body to recognize fullness.

- Make sure you eat slowly, putting your fork down between bites.

- Wait 10–15 minutes before going for something sweet or for second helpings. If you really want second helpings, ask yourself 'How will this make me feel in half an hour?' Will you feel bloated and stuffed? Do you want to go to sleep feeling like that? If the answer is that you are simply still hungry, have more vegetables and a little protein.

Those Stressy Habits Resolved

- Put some lavender or geranium essential oil into an oil burner while you cook to help you relax – also good in the bedroom when preparing for sleep.

- If you're having wine with dinner, choose sulphate-free – preferably organic – and stick to a small glass.

- If you are a TV eater, dinner away from the box might take time to get used to. Try and start with one or two nights a week and gradually build up to every night.

- Once you have finished, breathe, chat or listen to the others for at least 10 minutes before opting for a second helping or for pudding. This will give your body enough time to register satiety and fullness.

- If you fancy something sweet, try some seasonal fruit with Greek yoghurt or a square or two of dark chocolate (unless chocolate keeps you awake).

Making the Balance Work for You		
Stressy Evening	**Finding Your Balance**	**De-Stress Success**
Working late, no time to cook	Step away from the crisps and breathe. If this happens regularly, one-pot weekend cooking can be frozen into batches to take out on mornings you know you will be working late and reheated before serving with a large salad.	See stew and soup recipes on page 100. Curried and salsa-based dishes freeze particularly well as do chilli mince or bean stews. These can be taken out on mornings you know you will be late, so you have something that only needs heating when you get home.
Sunday night take-away	No need to feel like you're missing out if everyone is ordering take-aways. Try and stick to no more than one night a fortnight if you can, as they become more of a treat and as preparing your own food becomes easier.	See list above for the healthiest take-away options. If you can, ask what oil is used for frying – ghee, coconut or palm oil are best – and check that it is changed daily.

After work drinks – forgot to eat	If you know you're going out at night, eat a mid-afternoon snack just before. Make sure it includes some healthy fats and protein – Brazil nuts or celery with nut butter, a chunk of goat's cheese with cucumber or carrot sticks and tzatziki dip – to help slow the absorption of alcohol.	If you're drinking after work and there are nibbles on offer everywhere, stick to olives. They contain beneficial monounsaturated fatty acids that will help keep you satisfied longer. Be careful of too many nuts if they are roasted and salted; cooking nuts damages the omega oils.
Oops, I just downed 1,200 calories in one go at a dinner party	Be aware of any obligation you may feel to be polite and eat everything on your plate when out with friends. Above all, listen to your body. Avoid the bread basket, potato mountains and second helpings, and eat slowly, taking in the conversation so you stay in touch with your body's feelings of fullness and stop eating when you feel satisfied.	Remember, we evolved to eat a little less on some days, a bit more on others and occasionally, a lot. It's okay. If you ate a little more than usual last night, know your body will cope. The De-Stress Diet lifestyle essentials are designed as a scaffold to help your body through times like this without weight gain or adverse effects. Get back to the De-Stress Diet, relaxation and movement essentials and tell yourself that occasionally eating a lot of food – and in company – was one of our ancestors' leading lifestyle traits! Don't beat yourself up.

Lab Chat: Home Cooking

A study at the University at California found that putting together a home-cooked dinner takes on average only 10 minutes more of hands-on time than using mainly pre-packaged dishes.[20]

Troubleshooting: Dinner

These practical suggestions will help you deal with common evening obstacles that could sabotage your efforts.

PROBLEM: *You crave comfort carbs at night such as sweet foods and salty snacks.*

SOLUTION: Before you comfort eat, ask yourself 'What is this about?' Do you feel angry, tired or wired? Is there something – other than what you're about to eat – that might help more? If your comfort is sitting in front of the television and eating something numbing, think about other ways to soothe yourself. If you fancy food comfort in the form of creamy pasta or crisps, your body might simply be craving calming fats. Good fats such as avocado, a knob of butter, chopped nuts or pine nuts added to vegetables can help satisfy that urge and provide a feeling of calm without the excess salt, junk fats and blood-sugar spikes. If you feel wired and manic, your body may be craving comfort food simply to calm down. Try an Epsom or Himalayan salt bath before bed for immediate calm to your muscles and mind. Replace crisps with pumpkin or sunflower seeds, they are rich in tryptophan.

If you really are going to succumb to sweetness, choose a banana – they calm by helping GABA and serotonin levels. Wholemilk, plain yoghurt with cinnamon and coconut can also satisfy extreme cravings if you're weaning yourself off desserts. A little quality rock or sea salt added to dinner may support flagging adrenal glands (as long as you don't have high blood pressure) which could be making you crave salty snacks.

· ·

PROBLEM: *You go the gym after work and get home too late for cooking.*

SOLUTION: About an hour before you exercise, have a piece of fruit such as a pear, apple or cup of berries and some almonds or Brazil nuts to stabilize blood sugar so you don't get home famished afterwards. If you really must exercise on an empty stomach, have some coconut water before your workout to provide electrolytes and natural energy. Defrost a portion of ready-made stew or put on the slow cooker before you leave in the morning. Keep smoked salmon or mackerel in the fridge to make a simple salad, picking up a bag of salad greens in the day – both fish freeze well in packets and can be put out to defrost in the morning. Choose 'high-satiety' foods that don't upset body chemistry: a small portion of new potatoes in their skins is almost three times as satisfying as pasta, chips or rice and can stave off sweet cravings after a meal. Apples and oranges satisfy appetite better than cake, biscuits and ice cream.[21]

. . . .

PROBLEM: *You can't calm down before bed.*

SOLUTION: Have a 'tech amnesty' at least an hour before bed, as flashing images and light close to the face from laptops and phone screens affect melatonin production, which can make it harder to get to sleep. Supplement with magnesium and prioritize magnesium-rich foods for dinner when you're having a wired day: nuts, dark green leafy vegetables, carrots, avocado, fish, sunflower and sesame seeds, tahini, miso soup and tofu.

If you have long-term insomnia you may also find supplementation of 500–1,000mg of the amino acid taurine helpful alongside magnesium[22] (see page 127). This is found in fish, meat and milk so vegetarians may need to supplement it; the body can produce some but this may suffer in times of stress or low vitamin B_6 levels. Taurine and magnesium act like GABA, our brain's natural 'braking system', helping us switch off and fall asleep. These may be particularly helpful if overthinking or recurrent thoughts are getting in the way of sleep.

Use 'sleep teas' such as chamomile, valerian, hops, lemon balm, passionflower.

Make sure you get enough sunlight during the day for vitamin D needed for correct calcium and magnesium utilization, and ensure you eat plenty of sulphur foods on page 60 to ensure full vitamin D production.

If your brain just won't switch off, get into the habit of writing down persistent thoughts in a notebook or diary. Try a yoga nidra CD/audio download: this is the 'yoga of sleep' and is a guided full-body relaxation that works for many people who find it difficult to relax.

. . . .

PROBLEM: *You wake through the night because of baby/ neighbours/snoring partner.*

SOLUTION: Try to keep stress hormones as low as possible: stay in bed when you can and keep the lights off. Rather than lying there gnashing your teeth and getting frustrated, revel in the fact that you are in a warm, soft, comfy place with no pressure and the opportunity to appreciate it because you are awake – works for Charlotte when she can't get back to sleep after feeding her baby. Listen to a meditation, breathing or yoga nidra CD or audio. Catch up with sleep when you can, for example with an afternoon power nap next day. Some lavender drops on your pillow can help you stay calm and more likely to drop off. Use meditation and restorative yoga postures at any time possible during the day when you can't quite seem to get enough sleep.

PROBLEM: *You wake suddenly in the small hours.*

SOLUTION: Blood-sugar highs and lows throughout the day mean you can't sustain levels throughout the night causing a hypoglycaemic crash around 4 a.m. This results in an adrenaline surge that stops you slipping into a coma but can leave you suddenly awake, fearful and mind racing. Work on daytime stress and blood-sugar issues to get to the root cause. This advice can also apply to those who have disrupted sleep patterns caused by air travel or shift work. Have a bedtime snack – slow-release carbohydrate foods such as apples or oatcakes help to regulate blood-glucose levels throughout sleep. A few stalks of celery also calm the nervous system effectively. Turn the alarm clock to face other way. Seeing the time switches on your sympathetic nervous system and could lead to more anxiety about the amount of sleep you're missing. Take long, slow breaths and imagine your body melting into the mattress…

Help for Your Specific Stress Suit

Our Stress Suits give us clues about both what we need and how we can fix it – particularly in the evening, when what we need can differ wildly from what we want…

	You may find that you…	Best Single Change You Could Make
Stressed and Wired	can't stop 'doing' and then just can't get to sleep	Make time to do a full 15-minute calming activity to retrain your nervous system and mind. Celery is a traditional sleep remedy, with studies showing that its active chemical, apigenin, relaxes the nervous system and lowers blood pressure.[23]
Stressed and Tired	feel shattered when you get home but then become awake around 9 p.m.	Aim for 8 hours' sleep nightly, prioritizing quality sleep. De-Stressing as much as possible during the day will naturally feed into better energy early evening, followed by natural sleep. Do a gentle early evening yoga practice.
Stressed and Cold	feel sluggish in the evening but still feel unrefreshed after sleep	Don't overheat your house or bedroom, so that you stay alert (but calm) until the time you fully prepare for bed. Use blackout curtains if needed to shut off night-time stimulation to the pineal gland from light.
Stressed and Bloated	bloat after dinner, feeling gassy in the evening	Ensure dinner is light enough to digest and mindfully eaten to ensure full absorption. Probiotics taken at night can work well overnight, aiding best immune-modulation and helping address root causes of gas. Lying-down yoga twists can help.
Stressed and Sore	notice that inflammatory conditions worsen with poor sleep	Stay away from the inflammatory and excitory sugars and remember that good-quality sleep means your immune system has the chance to clean up the day's invaders and repair areas of inflammation.
Stressed and Demotivated	sleep and sleep and sleep at the weekends	This might pay back a little of your sleep debt but ultimately resets your sleep cycles, making it harder to get up on Monday morning. Try to change your perception so you can recognize the benefits of getting more sleep through the week and, therefore, more weekend activity time.

Stressed and Hormonal	notice that any of the above get worse before a period or menopausally	Prioritize De-Stress daily activities and make the evening time a sanctuary, particularly if you are used to clearing up and looking after others. Stay aware of how your breathing patterns signal when you are stressed.

Chapter 9

STRESS-FREE DRINKS AND SNACKS

People often underestimate the amount of extra food, excess sugar, unhealthy fats and chemicals that sneak into their diets as drinks and snacks. Our ancestors would have had the odd bit of fruit, some nuts and only water to drink, and while the occasional 'treat' is fine, craving cycles and a need to turn constantly to snacks or sugary drinks is a sign that your main meals and lifestyle are not supporting your energy needs. This chapter will help you move away from consuming mindless snacks and drinks.

The De-Stress Diet favours more sustaining meals over the 'little and often' ethos that has become popular recently and never gives the body the chance to experience true hunger. Less snacking means feeling liberated from a sense that food is controlling you, especially when this is supported by the De-Stress lifestyle changes that bring natural calm.

A recent study looking at American food habits in the last 30 years found that the amount of times people ate in a day rose from 3.8 to 4.9.[1] During that time obesity rates doubled for adults and tripled for children. The hormone ghrelin, which sets off hunger and a rumbling tummy, has been shown to be lower after meals containing fats and/or protein, while meals based on carbohydrates don't satisfy hunger in the same way and cause ghrelin to rise again quickly afterwards.[2] As high-carb, low-fat diets have been the mainstay of weight-loss recommendations for decades, this explains the continual need for snacking that has also become part of that picture. The advice to snack between meals shouldn't be necessary if healthy fats and proteins are included in main meals. On the De-Stress Diet you will ideally be sustained by meals alone, but stress and restrictions on the timing of your meals —for example, if you need to leave longer than around 4 hours between meals – can mean you need a well-timed and chosen snack. For most of us, 4 p.m. usually signals a natural energy lull, when tired adrenal glands and the related blood-sugar low can struggle to make the metabolic changes that move the body systems towards evening recovery over daytime activity mode. The right snack can pre-empt this and tide you through a journey home from work, keeping energy stable so you make good dinner choices. The same can be said of mid-morning if your breakfast and lunch times are too far apart.

De-Stress Snack Rules

The De-Stress Diet will help you crave less. By supporting your bio-chemistry, changing habits won't mean relying on willpower alone. This can be challenging as you move away from craving cycles, but these healthy snack guidelines can help the transition:

- Identify the healthiest snacks that you like, and have them on hand where you might need them.

- Don't be fooled by marketing ploys: 23 almonds contain a quarter-teaspoon of sugar compared to one low-fat 'health' bar based on a 'slimming' cereal which has around 2 teaspoons, as well as a whole host of additives.

- Don't keep problem snacks in the house. This includes diet sodas or whatever you are drawn to for that hit, unless you are one of those unusual types who can have a tub of ice-cream in the freezer and forget that it's there.

- If you feel intense hunger between meals or need to leave longer than 4–5 hours before your next meal, have a savoury snack that contains protein, such as almonds, to sate the driving hunger signals but not fuel a sweet tooth.

- If baking is one of your De-Stress activities, focus on savoury goods (coconut or almond flours are good grain substitutes) and, if sweet, use grated carrot or beetroot, cinnamon, coconut, dried fruit, apple puree or some xylitol to sweeten.

- Consider a cinnamon or fenugreek supplement to help sensitize your cells to insulin and support this time of withdrawal from snacking, especially if you are finding reducing sugar particularly difficult.

Best Snack Choices

The following are the best snacks for energy, before exercise to ensure good fuel supplies or even as beginner's breakfasts to ease into a new morning routine:

De-Stress Trail Mix

Equal portions of any of the following:

- raw, unsalted nuts – choose and vary almonds, Brazils, hazelnuts, walnuts, pecans
- pumpkin and sunflower seeds
- dried, unsweetened coconut
- unsulphured dried apricots, apple or mango – chopped to satisfy sweet cravings
- goji berries (reputed to support the adrenal glands)
- raw cocoa nibs can satisfy a chocolate craving and provide anti-oxidant polyphenols

Mix and store in an airtight container. A handful is a daily portion.

Vegetable Sticks

Slice any raw vegetables that you like for crunch – celery, carrots, red peppers, cucumber, and fennel all provide different nutrients. These can be stored in water with a little lemon juice for freshness and dipped in hummus, nut butters, mashed avocado or mackerel paté.

Hearty Smoothie

Blend the following:

- ½ large avocado
- ½ tin coconut milk (or make up 200ml from a coconut block)
- 200ml freshly squeezed apple juice or water, or a mix of the two
- 1 cup berries – strawberries, blueberries, raspberries or mixture (can be defrosted from frozen or blended while still partially frozen)

Less liquid will make more like a mousse, water can be added.
Add optional ground almonds, whey, pea or hemp protein for a sports blend or breakfast choice.

How Sugar Masquerades in Food Labels

Sugar is sugar, and saying it is 'natural' or organic does not change its effects in the body – if it tastes sweet, it is.[3] Moreover, increased exercise is no reason to increase sugar intake. Higher activity means a higher need for protective antioxidants, and sugar increases this need even more, raising inflammatory pathways and impeding muscle performance and strength. Sports nutrition products can be high in sugars, when natural fruits and nuts are far more suited to fuelling exercise. Manufacturers have many ways of fooling us about the sugar content of foods – see the list of hidden sugars below, often seen in fruit 'flavoured' products, even the very 'natural', organic ones:

- agave syrup
- barley malt
- brown rice syrup
- brown sugar

- cane juice
- corn sweetener
- corn syrup
- date sugar
- demerara sugar
- dextrin
- dextrose
- fructose (from fruits and grains)
- fruit juice concentrate
- galactose (from milk)
- glucose
- granulated sugar
- high-fructose corn syrup
- honey
- invert sugar
- lactose (from milk)
- malted barley
- maltodextrin
- maltose
- mannitol, sorbitol, xylitol
- maple syrup
- microcrystalline cellulose
- molasses
- polydextrose
- raisin juice
- raw sugar
- sucrose
- unrefined sugar
- white sugar

Natural Sugars

Natural fruit sugars like fructose (sugar from fruit) and date sugar are not better because they appear to come from plants (all sugars do, except lactose in milk). They are still processed, and fructose is more difficult than sucrose (table sugar) for our bodies to process.[4] Although causing less of a rise in blood-sugar, fructose can raise blood triglycerides (fats) and rob the liver of energy when it's eaten outside the safe package of a whole fruit. High Fructose Corn Syrup (HFCS) is a major sweetener in processed foods in the US and has been linked to the rise in obesity.[5] Honey is the only sugar source our ancestors would have eaten, but very occasionally. It has a lower Glycaemic Index than refined sugar, but it is still high in fructose, so use it sparingly and pay a little more if you can for antibacterial Manuka to help you use less.

Artificial Sweeteners

Sweeteners are often added to products to be able to label them as 'diet' or 'low sugar' but this isn't a healthier option. The science and evidence remain unclear about sweeteners, but remember these are designed to cause a response in the brain, the results of which remain inconclusive. Aspartame, for instance, a common sweetener for 'diet' products, sweets and soft drinks (as brands Nutrasweet and Equal), has recently been shown to raise glucose levels in people with diabetes.[6]

Sweeteners aren't 'free calories', they come with a price, keeping a sweet tooth and cravings alive, and are often present in highly processed foods that upset our biochemistry – much better to save a sweet taste and occasionally go for a better quality chocolate or pudding as a treat. When our brains are told we have eaten something sweet but then don't receive the calories, this can set up an imbalanced feedback loop of appetite regulation, leaving us with raised appetite.[7] If you use sugar or sweeteners in tea or coffee, don't find substitutes, wean yourself off – a sweet tooth is quickly changed.

> **DSD Tip**
> Anything over 10g of sugar per 100g on a label is a lot, and with a processed food that can equate to sugars that raise blood sugar and turn to fat. A can of a sweet fizzy drink has around 4 teaspoons of sugar.[8]

Not So 'Good for You'

Some food and drinks are smartly marketed as the healthy option, but aren't always so. When you have been on the De-Stress Diet for a few weeks you may begin to tune into how sweet these foods taste and how they make you feel; probably more depleted and not quite as satisfied as you had expected. Be wary of the following foods which may be masquerading as healthy (or at least not obviously unhealthy):

- **Vitamin or Fruit 'Waters'** – not just fruit juice and water, these are usually very high in sugar even though will often say 'all natural' on the label.

- **Diet sodas** – have been shown to significantly increase waistlines in humans.[9]

- **Fruit juices** especially from concentrate, but imagine how much fruit – without fibre – is needed to make just one glass. Commercial orange juice can have more sugar than the equivalent volume of cola. Have the odd glass of freshly squeezed juice and dilute by up to 50 per cent with water to reduce the sugar and cost. High fruit-juice intake has shown to be related to obesity, and the benefits of vitamin C and antioxidants are outweighed by the sugar content. Better to choose the whole fruit instead.

- **Commercial smoothies**, even those with 'no added sugar' still pack a punch of fructose or sugar from fruit. These can be preferable to juice as they include more fibre, but check the label for added sugars and limit your intake to treats only, choosing dark fruits and berries for best blood-sugar balance.

- **Drinks** like hot chocolate but also mocha coffees, iced coffee drinks and flavoured coffees with added syrups and hidden sugars.

- **Processed, commercial cereals** are not a good snack choice. Even if it says 'added fibre' on the packet, this is often harsh insoluble bran fibre which can irritate the gut. So-called slimming cereals often have a high Glycaemic Index (releasing their sugars too quickly) and the low-fat claims that come with the marketing mean they can be like eating rather unsatisfying air.

- **'Healthy' snack bars** of the slimming variety are generally low on the fat and protein which might satisfy your appetite, and often high in sugar. Their lightness and sweetness say it all: this will not fill you up.

- **Dried fruit** can be a useful dietary component if used sparingly and seen as the concentrated sugar source that it is. Imagine the sugar in one grape – this amount is present in one raisin in a concentrated package. Dates are the worst choice as their sugars hit the bloodstream as fast as pure glucose. See 'Best Sweet Alternatives' below.

DSD Tip
Sugary drinks have been shown to dull the palate and create a preference for sweet foods in just 2 weeks; always better to choose water, herbal or green tea.[10]

Best Sweet Alternatives

One of the objects of the De-Stress Diet is to reduce habitual sweet tastes in your diet. The following occasional healthy treat can be a halfway house to giving in entirely on those more challenging or stressful days. Buy the best quality when you plan to eat something sweet, and enjoy it without guilt:

- Dried mango, apricots, figs, prunes, apples – buy unsweetened and 'unsulphured' without the preservative sulphur dioxide, which can cause digestive discomfort.

- Stewed apples and plums sweetened with a little honey.

- Baked apples – easy to add honey, cinnamon and then keep for later as delicious sliced treats.

- Healthy snack bars – many of these are incredibly sweet as they are based on high-sugar dates (it is their syrupy stickiness that glues the bar together). Look for those with nuts and the least amounts of the sugars listed earlier in this chapter (see pages 142–43); beware the bar with a sugar source high up on the list. We have some suggestions at de-stressyourlife.com

- Oat-based biscuits or flapjacks can be the best occasional choice if you're going to succumb to the sugar/grain combination, as they release their sugars slowly.

- If you're having the odd fruit-based pudding, choose a little cream over custard or ice-cream, as this is sweetened only by the natural lactose present in dairy.

Chocolate

With a poll of 1,965 people showing some women rate chocolate above sex, and men above a spin in a sports car,[11] it is with caution that we tell you to reduce your intake. Chocolate is rich in anti-inflammatory and heart-protective polyphenol antioxidants also found in wine or green tea, but always has some form of sugar added.[12] Don't be fooled by talk of 'natural sugars', chocolate is bitter and if it's sweet contains sugar. Choose small amounts of high-quality chocolate to take advantage of the 'happy chemical' beta-endorphins which it helps the brain produce. But don't kid yourself: much of this effect is from the sugar and fat combination.[13]

Chocolate Guidelines

- A 40g or so small bar of dark chocolate every few days is fine, flavoured with mint or orange oil, nuts, chilli or other spices. One study showed that 40g a day of dark chocolate helped people cope with stress.[14]

- A 40g bar of milk chocolate will contain not only dairy, but also as much as 7 teaspoons of sugar compared to a 3-teaspoon average for the same weight of 70 per cent cocoa dark chocolate.

- 5 or 6 dark chocolate-covered Brazil nuts have more of the nut protein present so come with more flavour and satisfaction.

- Pay more and buy less. Favouring quality over quantity can make you more of a healthy connoisseur than an unhealthy sugar addict.

- Raw chocolate has become popular because, unlike commercial preparations, the beans aren't roasted, retaining much higher levels of antioxidants, less agitating caffeine effect and is often made with coconut cream instead of dairy.

Fruit

Our ancestors ate fruit, which of course seems natural and healthy. Our recommendations to eat 2–3 portions of fruit maximum a day can help keep your diet mainly savoury and reduce the likelihood of excess dietary sugar converting to fat. Apples and berries are particularly good fruit choices as these blunt the rise of digested sugars after a meal. This makes them good choices if you are weaning off a dessert habit, but pick berries if you tend towards bloating as apples (and potentially other fruit) easily ferment if eaten straight after protein. Apples, apricots, cherries, oranges, plums (and also carrots) contain the soluble fibre pectin, which satisfies appetite by holding food in the stomach for longer. Pectin has also been shown to limit the amount of fat your cells can absorb to help curb damage from meals high in saturated fat. Grapes, mangoes, dried apricots, dried figs, dates, raisins, watermelon and bananas are high in sugar, particularly fructose, so the least healthy choices – but still a better occasional choice than an artificial sugar hit if you're struggling with sweet cravings.

Nuts and Seeds

Nuts may be high in anti-nutrients (nature is full of them!) but part of our hunter-gatherer ancestors' diets, so it is believed that we are more adapted to the lectins they contain. They provide crucial protein for vegetarians (and especially vegans), soluble fibre, minerals and essential oils. They contain immune-modulating properties, especially almonds eaten with their skin, and those who include nuts in their diet tend to have better weight management.[15] Again, almonds in particular provide excellent appetite satisfaction.[16] Nuts also have a neutral acid–alkaline balance, making them a better source of starchy carbohydrates than grains.

Hydration

Like snacks, drinks have become a massive industry, and yet it is easy to be dehydrated if we take in too little water through the most natural route: from whole vegetables and fruits. Sugary drinks, including those sold as 'vitamin' drinks and sports drinks, also contribute to obesity and blood-sugar imbalances.

Insufficient hydration can have an impact on all aspects of health. Bloating can be one side effect as your body holds on to the little it is receiving, affecting digestion and detoxification. Hydration is crucial during exercise for endurance and coordination, and low levels can result in histamine production, triggering inflammation. Dehydrated muscle performs badly and is more prone to injury.

Having said that, the '2 litres a day' message is now being refuted in many scientific corners, with a preference for drinking when thirsty and hydrating from fluid- and mineral-rich vegetables and fruits.[17] This helps avoid the mineral loss and strain on our kidneys that too much water alone can bring. Too high a water intake can produce hyponatremia or low sodium levels in the blood, and can lead to symptoms of confusion, fatigue, irritability and muscle cramps – worth checking out with your GP if you have been drinking over 2 litres of water a day.

When you are generally hydrated with good mineral balances, it is easier to connect to your natural thirst mechanism. This kicks in when we lose about 1–2 per cent of our body's water (mild dehydration) and will vary according to how much exercise you are doing and how hot and/or dry your environment is; air-conditioning and air travel definitely qualify as dehydrating. Stress and disordered breathing patterns can also cause more moisture loss and, if over 2 per cent of normal water volume is lost, true dehydration with possible dry skin and loss of appetite occurs. Timing is crucial: many people drink too little water between meals, providing little liquid with which to produce digestive juices and keep the bowel hydrated. Not chewing enough prompts drinking with meals to lubricate food for swallowing, but this can dilute stomach acid, reducing digestive efficacy further. Make sure you drink water between meals, sip only a little with food.

Better Hydration Through Your Diet

Simply increasing the amount of water in a dehydrated body can be like watering a dry pot-plant: you see the water go straight through without being absorbed. Try these methods to help hydrate your body:

- Increase vegetable and fruit intake. Fruits and veg contain potassium and sugars that help the water they contain enter cells more easily than water alone, while soluble fibre hydrates the bowel. The soups and stews we recommend in Chapter 6 are particularly effective.

- If your diet has been low in fruit and veg, high in caffeine and added stress, dehydration-related symptoms such as constipation, headaches and dry skin may have been the result. Increase your liquid intake slowly, substituting sugary snacks for 2 glasses of half-apple juice (freshly pressed 'cloudy' version), half-water for the first few weeks of the plan, then tapering off to replace with water and the recommended fluids.

- Drink warm or hot water, especially with meals – chilled water takes energy away from digestion to heat up and may cause muscular contractions at the shock.

- As an isotonic fluid, coconut water contains the same balance of minerals as our own blood plasma and can be helpful for replenishing stores lost during exercise.[18] It is a much better health choice than the very sugary commercial isotonic sports drinks available; Charlotte's athletic clients report it as good for performance and recovery.

- Drink filtered water with lemon juice for alkalizing with the fewest impurities; filter water at home and carry in a stainless steel or BPA-free plastic bottle for the day. Do not re-use soft plastic bottles. See more at de-stressyourlife.com

- Herbal teas are an excellent non-caffeinated way to hydrate, especially if you make your own from fresh mint, fennel seeds or fresh ginger and lemon. Add cinnamon to sweeten and a tiny bit of honey only as you are weaning yourself off sugar.

- Spice teas taste great and also supply the properties of the spices, especially when made without a teabag. A chai Indian tea mix typically includes any of the following in varying amounts: cardamom, cinnamon, ginger, fennel seeds, peppercorn, licorice and cloves. Make a simple blend to your taste, adding ¼ teaspoon per small mug of water and drink the spices.

- Rooibush or redbush tea is non-caffeinated African tea that is the best substitute for the normal 'cuppa'. It comes in flavoured versions, too, like vanilla, chai and Earl Grey.

Caffeine

Anthropologists believe that we have been imbibing caffeine in low levels in green tea since the Stone Age.[19] It is an extremely reliable drug, delivering a quick jolt to your central nervous system for the increased wakefulness, mental acuity, alertness and focus that make it so attractive. But this is stealing a quick fix; it doesn't remove the need for rest, just masks the sensations of tiredness. As a stimulant caffeine directly tells the pituitary gland to tell the adrenal glands to produce adrenaline, so energizing but also raising sugar- and fat-storing insulin levels.[20] The reliance on this unnatural energy comes from the fact that it binds to adenosine receptors in the brain, keeping these energy-stimulators revved up and stopping tendencies for the blood vessels to dilate and feel oxygenated and sleepy as we might do before bed. This is not good pre-sleep, and if you consider that our bodies are preparing these retiring processes from 4 p.m. onwards (even though we switch on those lights and keep going), caffeine is definitely not advised past around 2–3 p.m.

When broken down, caffeine creates three chemicals. First, paraxanthine, which breaks down fats but then leaves them dangerously floating round the bloodstream.[21] Second, theobromine, the same chemical from which chocolate gets its Latin name *theobroma*, which causes vasodilation, increasing oxygen and nutrient flow to the muscles and brain (the reason many sportspeople use caffeine before training). Third, theophylline relaxes smooth muscle, which has been linked to its natural laxative properties (but caffeine can also irritate the gut to the same effect). Caffeine is also thermogenic, which means it increases the body's heat and metabolic action, so small amounts without sugar can help increase fat-burning rather than storage and sate appetite. Studies have consistently failed to show that caffeine causes dehydration in moderate amounts,[22] but its diuretic effects in levels higher than a few cups a day may tell, especially if it's your only fluid source.

Caffeine in tea, coffee, chocolate, colas and some energy drinks is best avoided if you feel it is making you more stressed. For some of us, though, high-quality coffee or tea can provide a healthy lift if kept to 2 cups maximum a day, for example one after breakfast and/ or lunch.[23] If you're having a shop-bought coffee ask for a single shot only so as not to over-stimulate your system. If you're used to having a cup of coffee or tea before breakfast, save this until you have food in your stomach. Coffee on an empty stomach and low blood sugar causes a greater surge in adrenaline in response to the caffeine, and this high could come with a sudden crash later. Caffeine can affect mineral absorption from a meal, so is not a good idea alongside grains or beans.

Lowering Caffeine Slowly

Like most drugs, physical dependency on caffeine comes from the dopamine 'reward high' it produces.[24] That's why caffeine withdrawal can lead to headaches, fatigue, moodiness and constipation. Symptoms generally occur after 12 hours without, peak after 24–48 hours and last up to a week. Knowing this helps to see the reactions for what they are, and also to plan how to manage withdrawal alongside sugar reduction. Aim to get high caffeine levels down to 2 cups a day, after food. But if you also have lots of sugar in your diet, prioritize lowering sugar intake first and taper off your caffeine slowly so that you don't see sugar craving worsen before you have increased natural energy levels. Fewer stimulants can eventually mean fewer sugar cravings, but this can take weeks to settle. Include De-Stress lifestyle issues to help calm your nervous system as you cut down.

DSD Tip

Licorice tea is the best alternative for those who have become Stressed and Tired and struggle to maintain natural energy without stimulants. It keeps cortisol circulating when it is low,[25] so it's good for a natural energy boost in the morning – but not past early afternoon. This effect is so good though, that licorice tea is contra-indicated for those with high blood pressure.[26] Commercial blends in tea bags are readily available, or licorice root flakes can be added to water or herbal tea.

Caffeine withdrawal can come with extreme energy slumps as your brain chemistry re-sensitizes to using its own natural energy. Plan for this and reduce on a Friday to give yourself a seriously laid-back weekend, using the advice in Chapter 11 to support you. Prioritize bringing down any sugar or sweeteners in tea or coffee first, replacing with cinnamon if this suits you. If yours is the Stressed and Wired Suit, try to use caffeine only as an occasional treat when you really need it.

Theobromine and theophylline are still present in decaffeinated drinks, so will create some stimulation. Choose good-quality water-filtered decaf if you're choosing this option, but better stick to green tea or herbal teas. Tea and coffee can be sprayed with huge amounts of chemicals, so choose organic or use green tea as a replacement for stronger black tea and coffee.

DSD Tip

Green tea is a great replacement for stronger black tea and coffee – like all tea, it has high levels of protective antioxidant catechins[27] which counter the over-stimulating effects of the small amount of caffeine present.[28] Try different brands and varieties, only brew for 30 seconds to avoid a bitter taste, and try chai and other flavoured versions if you are not keen at first. The Japanese *Genmaicha* and *Sencha* varieties are nutritious and delicious. Green tea also contains a substance called L-Theanine, known to have calming effects on body and mind. Taken in concentrated form in supplements, it may help reduce mental and physical stress and increase mental focus.[29]

How Much Caffeine Are You Getting?

About 200–300mg daily caffeine is generally recommended as the safe upper limit to help prevent the related insomnia, anxiety, nausea and accelerated heart rate that comes with over-stimulation. When you also consider that a 'grande'-sized coffee from a well-known High Street coffee chain has as much as 350mg per cup, you can suddenly see why there are so many highly agitated folk about. For some, though, symptoms can be set off even by a weak cup of tea, so monitor your own reactions.

300mg caffeine roughly equates to:

- 4 average cups or 3 average-sized mugs of instant coffee
- 3 average cups of brewed coffee
- 6 average cups of tea
- 8 cans of regular cola drinks
- 4 cans of 'energy drinks'
- 400g (8 standard 50g bars) of plain chocolate

Individual intakes average at:[30]

- Average cup of instant coffee – 75mg

- Average mug of coffee – 100mg

- Average cup of brewed coffee – 100mg

- Average cup of tea – 50mg

- Regular cola drink – up to 40mg

- Regular energy drink – up to 80mg

- Plain bar of chocolate – up to 50mg. Caffeine in milk chocolate is about half that in plain chocolate

Alcohol

Red wine contains protective antioxidants from a substance called resveratrol, found in red grape skins in much higher amounts than any other food. Less than two units a day of red wine has indeed been shown to be a contributory component in lowering heart disease and obesity risk,[31] and was a prominent feature of the healthiest Mediterranean diet of Crete,[32] where it was estimated to add a year to life expectancy when combined with the other longevity components such as plenty of vegetables, fruit, olive oil and garlic. But red wine is also an immediate sugar source and, for the Cretans, was always drunk with food, thus reducing its blood-sugar-raising effects.

Straying above the recommended 14 weekly units for women and 21 for men can soon negate these benefits, especially if you're clocking them all up on a Friday night, putting dangerous pressure on your liver. Remember, one unit is one 175ml glass of wine, not a large half-bottle glassful. It is not only binge-drinking but also that continual drip-feeding of daily alcohol to amounts above healthy limits that has been shown to increase risks of breast cancer, heart disease, diabetes and osteoporosis,[33] as well as damaging memory and reaction times.[34]

As a sugar source, alcohol has the same effects as any other, raising insulin and turning on fat storage by increasing fatty deposits in the liver.

The ethanol that causes intoxication is, by its very definition, toxic to the body and causes damage to all the liver's detoxification pathways. The liver works overtime to eject it, but the alcohol itself depletes the very substances needed to speed it out of the body, especially those required for energy and dealing with stress and blood-sugar balance, such as B vitamins, vitamin C, magnesium, zinc and chromium.

For many, alcohol may seem essential for 'switching off'. This is because its first response is to relax us by heightening the relaxing brain chemical GABA (gamma-amino butyric acid), our body's natural control mechanism for managing stress and nervous tension.[35,36] Sounds great, right? But this becomes a cycle where the brain starts to need alcohol to pick up the GABA and without it we can then become tense, anxious and unable to sleep. Using alcohol to help sleep is a false economy: the GABA rush does stupefy and relax at first, but then lowered levels throughout the night can impair sleep and jolt you awake in the small hours.

Reducing how much alcohol you drink can result in a phase where less GABA (and also dopamine) is available to the brain and you may feel agitation, anxiety and/or nervousness, while your brain gets sensitized to accessing its own GABA stores again. This can be difficult, especially for Stressed and Demotivated types, but it is crucial at this stage not to turn to other sugar sources to replace this effect and 'normalize'. That simply replaces one addictive cycle with another. Women may also experience more alcohol cravings premenstrually, as will anyone during times of stress, as the body's attempt to self-medicate.

De-Stress Guidelines for Alcohol

- If having a glass of wine with a meal several times a week is your treat, stick to that and avoid other sugar sources.

- Quality is key: spend more and buy less to become a connoisseur rather than a guzzler. You can even encourage your friends to do the same. The deeper the red, the higher the antioxidant count, with the best amounts seen in Merlot, Cabernet Sauvignon and

Chianti grapes. Rioja and Pinot Noir are in the middle, and the least benefit comes from Côtes du Rhône.

- Champagne or dry white wines contain less sugar than sweeter red or white wines; they are the best choice for those wanting the occasional celebratory drink while staying off sweet tastes.

- Gin or vodka with soda and a twist of lime are the best low-sugar choices, providing water for hydration and avoiding the problem sugars or sweeteners in mixers. Whisky, vodka, gin and rum have little sugar when drunk on their own, so switch to an occasional shot on the rocks.

- Beers, dessert wines, fortified wines (e. g. sherry, port), sweet wines and brandy all have high sugar content, so avoid them.

- Grain-based alcohols like beer, ales and vodka may affect those with grain intolerance.

- For everyone, good liver support is essential when reducing any addictive cycles. See pages 60 and 81 in the 6-Week Plan and ensure good hydration. A daily 1,000–2,000mg vitamin C is recommended by many nutritional therapists and naturopaths to help curb cravings and assist the liver in detoxifying alcohol.

See de-stressyourlife.com for a chart to help identify and reduce alcohol intake.

Social Lubrication

Britain is a nation of drinkers, and many people can feel extreme social pressure from friends and work colleagues not to appear 'boring' or different. Some people can be threatened when others reduce how much they drink or give up alcohol altogether, but a growing number of us are doing so, especially as we hit our late thirties and beyond and the hangovers get worse. Learning to go out without drinking to excess is a skill to be learned like any other, a reconditioning that takes practice but ultimately leads to feeling more yourself and sparing yourself the hideous aftermaths.

Consider whether you have a tendency to drink alone to numb yourself or combat 'bad stress'. Use the recommendations beginning on page 195 to help find alternative ways to relax, cope and move away from these negative coping patterns. Never drink on an empty stomach and always ensure you have good protein before a drink to curb blood-sugar spikes and help detoxify the alcohol. Eggs are especially good as they contain high levels of cysteine, a sulphur amino acid that helps break down alcohol – this is the reason they are an age-old hangover cure in many cultures. Sulphur is necessary for the liver detoxification pathway that disables alcohol; see the foods listed on page 60 to include in meals before, during and after drinking. Taking 500mg vitamin C and the liver-support supplements on page 68 before, during and after drinking can help limit the damage. This is not a free ticket to drink plenty, but a measure to allow a treat to harm you the least.

Avoiding friends or situations that revolve around alcohol can help while you change the biochemical effects, but is ultimately avoiding the problem. If you're out to dinner or in the pub chatting, pay attention to how much you are drinking. It is easy to keep knocking back a newly filled glass, especially in a culture where drinking more is lauded. Alternate alcohol with sparkling water with lemon (not sugary soft drinks or juice), to both support your liver and reduce alcohol intake. Learn to say no and not be pressured. It is your choice to drink or not, and not appropriate for others to badger, cajole or bully you into having more than you want; that is a form of social stress and if it's in your life it needs to be nipped in the bud with an assertive 'no thanks'.

If you drink to any level reaching near alcoholism (consult your GP to define this), do not give up alcohol suddenly as that can be very dangerous. Safe withdrawal is known as *tapering* and should be done under the supervision of a medical professional.

Snacks and Drinks by Stress Suit

	You may find that you...	Best single change you could make
Stressed and Wired	rely on a barrage of sugar, caffeine and/or alcohol to stay 'up'	Learn to view energy levels differently, allowing yourself to rest when your body and brain need recovery, including backing off the stimulants systematically and noting symptoms.
Stressed and Tired	can't make it to the next meal without craving something sweet	Use the 6-Week Plan to explore when you might need a well-chosen snack to level out long-term blood-sugar imbalances. Use cinnamon in food and teas to break craving cycles. Give up caffeine systematically so you do not turn to sugar instead. Use licorice tea to naturally energize.
Stressed and Cold	don't quite feel satisfied after meals and, although bloated, still want more	Drink a cup of strong peppermint tea (leave the teabag in to brew), about 20 minutes before eating a meal. Peppermint stimulates the production of both stomach acid and bile from the liver to get the best metabolic effect from your food.
Stressed and Bloated	end up snacking later as you avoid larger meals, especially when stressed	Avoid drinking an hour either side of meals, except the odd sip with food. Also avoid eating fruit after dense protein, as it may ferment and cause gas. Mix dried mint, ginger, cumin and fennel seeds for a post-meal digestive tea.
Stressed and Sore	aren't sure what's going on, you just seem so reactive to stress and different foods	Ensure good hydration levels, reduce sugars and caffeine and see digestive measures; all for preventing inflammation (pages 34–35). Add turmeric to spice tea mix and choose green tea as a mild caffeine source.
Stressed and Demotivated	end up eating sugar or comfort foods for no good reason, even when you know you 'shouldn't'	Find the right treats for you. The dark chocolate suggestion on page 148 might be the right thing for the moment, while you address other aspects of your diet; knowing you'll have that treat can help you resist others. Reduce caffeine, which may raise cortisol and reduce DHEA.
Stressed and Hormonal	want more sugar before your period	Snack on nuts if needed to provide soluble fibre, B vitamins and zinc for good hormone balance. 'Detox' teas can be a quick and easy extra liver support. Prioritize reducing alcohol, as it can raise oestrogen and is known to be a prominent breast cancer risk – none is best.

Part 3
THE DE-STRESS LIFESTYLE

Chapter 10

THE NEW MIND–BODY MOVEMENT

If you asked primal man to undertake some of today's exercise regimes, he may have looked at you as though you had just dropped your loincloth. Too many long, drawn-out periods of intense running or repetitive movements on machines would have exhausted his energy, perhaps injured him and put so much stress on his system that there would have been no vitality for life's duties, such as finding dinner or running away from predators dead set on making his family *their* next meal. Today we don't have such problems, and physical threats are a rarity in our cushioned lives. But emotional and psychological ones aren't – they don't get resolved as easily and they come with the same biological responses. For our stressful lifestyles, exercise is essential because it provides the activity our bodies need to burn off the hormones that flood our systems during the 'fight or flight' response. The glucose, insulin, adrenaline and cortisol that are mobilized in your body when you're under stress will promote fat storage if you sit at your desk, still and stewing with anxiety. By using the energy that stress generates, physical activity can reduce the physiological impact of stress on your body and make you feel better faster – even if what is causing your stress is still there. In fact, exercise has been shown to lower levels of circulating cortisol naturally in the body and be comparable – and in some cases better – for your mood than anti-depressants.[1] The more stressed you get, the more cortisol you release, the more fat you are likely to lay down. Not only does intelligent exercise make you feel better and increase your metabolic rate, it also makes it less likely that stress will create excess fat around your belly and more likely that, once lost, you can keep the weight off.[2]

The aim of the De-Stress Diet is to move away from hard, long workouts once or twice a week and think more in terms of significantly increasing the amount of activity in your daily life. We favour short, non-exhaustive movement sessions of varying intensities (in the form of general activity and structured exercise) done more often rather than long, energy-draining ones that most people only have the stamina to do once or twice a week.

An Emotional as Well as Physical Fix

Today's most enlightened fitness experts, including our fitness consultant Charlene Hutsebaut – a high-profile personal trainer who has designed the programmes in this chapter – are labelling notions of gruelling 'no-pain, no-gain' exercise as dated. These can leave us leaner in the short term but stressed and exhausted in the long term and more likely to lay down fat than build muscle. Studies, too, are now showing we don't have to exercise to exhaustion to get the bona-fide body and mood benefits of exercise: the strongest correlation between physical activity and psychological wellbeing is most pronounced with low to moderate physical activity. One review of exercise literature found that decreases in tension, depression, anger and confusion were associated with bouts of moderate activity exercise.[3]

We'll be urging you in this chapter to aim for exercise that provides you with both physical and emotional benefits. When we find exercise that works on our minds and makes us feel better, we're far more likely to stick to it. Old school trainers still suggest punishing regimes based on guilt and shame. But that rarely lasts unless you have a masochistic streak that gets a kick out of being bullied. Because excess amounts of the stress hormone cortisol can lead to muscle wasting, it can also lead to that sinewy, starved look that is often a tell-tale sign of an over-exercised, over-stressed and possibly under-nourished and under-hydrated body.

All this goes beyond simple endorphin rushes to a deeper sense of wellbeing and comfort in your skin. Unless exercise is helping you alleviate negative emotions, not creating them by stressing or exhausting your body, it won't work long term. And the best news? What makes you feel good will probably make you look good, too. That is certainly the case for the De-Stress Diet's exercise programme. We're not fans of preachy health advice, and exercise is one area where advice can sound condescending and unrealistic. This isn't an exercise guide for celebrities with plenty of time for getting into shape. It's a programme designed for the needs and life demands of real people.

The Best of Good Stressors

Remember the good stressors that make you stronger from Chapter 1? Exercise tops that list because the stress it puts on the body's cardiovascular, hormonal, muscular, and skeletal systems makes it come back stronger. All the benefits we know of exercise – increased metabolism and muscle tone, less tension and anxiety, more energy and glowing skin – can't happen without the little bits of good stress it puts on our bodies. These results come out of increased fitness and strength, and are signs of the body's adaptation to the regular episodes of good stress that exercise puts it under.

Here's how: your body has a natural equilibrium that it exists in day to day, which is the biological point at which it feels and behaves at its best. Too much ongoing, chronic stress can reset this ideal balance at a heightened rate, so the body expects more stress. Too much over-exercise has a similar effect. But the right kind of exercise, in regular bouts and alternated with regular periods of deep rest, challenges that equilibrium in a positive way. The heart rate goes up, muscle temperature and oxygen consumption rise but then get the chance to come down. Done regularly over time, this informs your body to get stronger and more efficient in response.

Naturally, your body's function peaks in your mid-thirties. From then on, basic fitness and aerobic capacity, as well as mobility, flexibility and strength, reduce. Ironically, this is usually the time in your life when stress may be at its worst – and rising – and when you need your strength, mobility and flexibility the most. By provoking an adaptation response to the regular stress of exercise – in any form – you can not only slow that progression down, you can build up your physiological strength and resources for dealing with stress during times when it increases in your life. For us, that is the real definition of 'fit' – not an airbrushed girl in a leotard – and thankfully, its by-product is usually a slim, toned, calm and comfortable body.

How We Evolved to Move

Some 2.4 million years ago, humans evolved from apes into the *Homo sapiens* species we are today, and for the majority of that time – about 84,000 generations – they lived as hunter-gatherers. Survival within that lifestyle required plenty of necessary movement and calorie-burning from finding food and water, social interaction, escaping from predators, building homes, washing clothes and carrying babies (believe it or not, the Bugaboo hadn't evolved yet). Though millions of years have passed since then, our bodies and their capabilities have remained genetically and physically the same, but our lifestyles have changed beyond recognition. Hunter-gatherers existed until about 10,000 years ago, which in evolutionary terms is, well, not long, and their lifestyles meant they weighed an average of 14 kilos less than we do today and expended about 400–600 calories more every day. This was mostly in the pursuit of food and precious calories, which also cultivated a respect for food eaten.

Today, we have ready-made food, people to build our homes, technology to do our work and, for most of us, daily toil involves more brain than body, exercising only our fingers at our keyboard while the rest of our body sits and sits and sits (the authors of this book are no exception: we obviously sat on our bottoms for long periods of time to write this book). In fact, according to a report in the *International*

Journal of Sports Medicine, the energy expenditure of a typical Westerner is about 38 per cent that of our primitive hunter-gatherer ancestors.[4] The bottom line is this: our bodies *love to move*. We evolved to move in many and varied ways. That means that if you think you hate exercise, it's probably because you haven't found something your body loves to do yet, and that you have got used to a level of inactivity that means the beginning of movement comes with a certain level of discomfort. We discuss this perception of pain or new feelings in Chapter 11, and how to move through the different levels of change that you might experience at the start.

So start slowly and give yourself the time and space to listen to your body as you build up strength and the ability to move and use oxygen efficiently. You will go through highs and lows, but keep at it and you will soon feel the benefits of exercise, such as increased wellbeing and calm and less tension.[5] Your body is built to move, and discomfort along the way is the release of habitual tension and reorganization of postural and muscular alignment. At least for a while, forget the circumference of your thighs (don't worry – thinner ones will come). Once you have felt the benefits of this programme, you will want to stay with it.

De-Stress Diet Fitness

We urge you to focus on the way you feel rather than the way you look during the first few weeks. By focusing on enjoying yourself, relieving stress and tension and increasing your energy and vitality, you're more likely to experience what most people who stick to exercise for many years know for sure – exercise makes you feel *amazing* and cope better with stress. This exercise programme works without exhausting you as long as you take the compulsory rest and recovery days. It's also designed for people with varied amounts of time and to be flexible so you can incorporate its elements into a programme that suits you. 'Suits you' here does not mean what your stress-driven mind can push you to do, but what your body truly needs on any given day or week: movement without exhaustion.

Quick Strength-training

One of the biggest factors influencing your metabolism is the amount of muscle in your body. That is because muscle burns more calories than fat. Even when we're resting, sitting and typing at a desk, our muscles are torching calories at a faster rate than our fat. We're not talking about bulky biceps or hamstrings but sleek, long muscles that come from the new, targeted fitness of smart – not hard – exercise. For years, exercise junkies have been obsessed with that magic number on the treadmill as the Holy Grail of fat loss: the amount of calories burned during your workout. But more and more exercise physiologists are realizing that not only is this long, hard slog exhausting and highly stressful for the body, it is also the least important or beneficial way to workout. What matters is your caloric *afterburn*, which is the amount of calories you burn *after* your workout. This is determined by the amount of muscle tone in your body. The right workout can elevate your Resting Metabolic Rate (RMR) for longer. This is optimized by activities that maximize muscle toning and *excess post-exercise oxygen consumption* (EPOC) – in other words, caloric afterburn.[6]

Lightweight training is one of the best ways of increasing muscle tone and EPOC, but doesn't have to be done on bulky machines. It can incorporate light weights or even your own body as the force. This is what Charlene's exercises here will do (and many yoga poses also provide this type of resistance). Plus, we'd prefer you didn't slog away for a whole hour. Studies have shown that people who do shorter, high-intensity toning exercise lose more fat and weight (especially around the middle),[7] and maintain more stable blood-sugar than those doing traditional aerobic exercise for hours on end.[8]

Determining Your Fitness Levels

The DSD exercise programme has an excellent variety of exercises meant to work the entire body. You may find you are stronger or more flexible on some exercises than others, so your 'fitness level' may vary between exercises.

The press-ups, for example, are divided into three levels for you. If you can do 12 press-ups at Level 1, then try some repetitions at Level 2. When you are confidently able to do 12 at Level 2, feel free to try several repetitions at Level 3. If you can do 12 at Level 3, then add more repetitions in a set.

All other exercises have a range of either sets or repetitions or both.

If you can do two sets of the lowest amount of repetitions comfortably, you are ready for Level 2. You can move to three sets of the lowest repetitions for several weeks, then move to three sets of the higher repetitions listed to Level 3. To keep challenging yourself after Level 3, add a fourth set. Another way to challenge yourself at any level is to add a heavier weight or larger cans in your hands in the exercises requiring lifting.

Level 1: 1–2 sets of 6–8 repetitions

Level 2: 2 sets of 8–12 repetitions

Level 3: 3 sets of 12–15 repetitions

Safe Exercise Technique

Mimic the sketches given, keeping a neutral spine. Imagine how a spine should look with all of its natural curves. Whether you are standing, squatting or bending at the waist, the spine should be neutral. If you are moving through a set and your back gets tired or the weights start to feel too heavy and cause you to come out of the proper neutral alignment, you are ready for a break. Stay at the level of sets and repetitions you are at until you feel stronger and can get through more repetitions with safe technique.

25-minute Strength-training Routine

If you are a beginner, aim to do this quick strength workout once or twice a week. If you are intermediate or advanced, go for up to four times a week, ensuring you have rest days between workouts.

Over-exercise is anathema to everything in the De-Stress Diet and can sabotage your weight-loss efforts by reflooding the system with stress hormones.

On the days you don't do this routine, make sure you maintain your activity levels with walking, swimming, social exercise and yoga (see the next Chapter).

This strength workout is designed to be done at home, in the park or gym, and we have given instructions for options in all three locations as well as some tweaks for different levels. It should take you around 25–30 minutes to complete depending on the number of sets you do. Beginners can start with the lower number of repetitions and work up towards 12; if intermediate or advanced you can do the higher amount, but everyone should complete all sets. The weight used for each set should challenge you without pain. Once you have completed this workout for 6 weeks, log onto de-stressyourlife.com to download another De-Stress Diet resistance workout based on your level and the time you have.

Warm-Up

Walking is one of the best ways to ease the body into increasing blood flow to the working muscles and stimulate natural lubrication at the joints. Below are other options. Remember to be conscious of your breathing as you move.

Home:

- March on the spot for 5 minutes

- Walk up and down stairs for 5 minutes

- 10 minutes easy on cardio machine (if you own one)

Gym:

- 10 minutes easy on cardio machine of your choice

- Ask a class instructor of any type if you can participate in his or her warm-up and then quietly leave to continue your own workout in another part of the gym – a good instructor shouldn't mind if you do this. Tell him or her you will stay near the door of the studio so that leaving doesn't disrupt the class.

Outside:
- Walk or gently jog around the park/block for 10 minutes.

Press-ups
3 sets of 6–12 repetitions

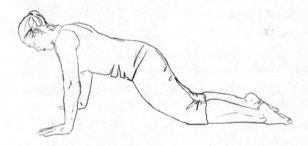

Level 1: Start on your hands and knees, hands just wider than shoulder-width apart, hips over knees.

Level 2: Start on your hands and knees, hands just wider than shoulder-width apart. Form a long board position from your shoulders to knees (imagine a straight line from your shoulders through hips to knees).

Level 3: Start on hands and toes – keep the body straight like a board from the shoulders to the toes.

All Levels
- Breathe in to bring your chest towards the floor or exercise mat, bending your elbows only to a 90-degree angle.
- Breathe out to come back up, straightening your elbows.
- Throughout the entire movement, keep your abdominal muscles gently tight by pulling your belly button towards your spine.
- Keep your shoulder blades in a neutral position (floating flat on the back/rib cage, down towards the hips).

- Lead with your chest, keeping your head and neck in line with your spine. The old school 'take your nose to the floor'... is not safe!
- Ideally you should be able to do three sets of between 6 and 12 press-ups at the level you have chosen, keeping your back in a neutral position.
- If you can do 12 of a level, then try some repetitions of the next level up.
- If you can do 12 of Level 3, then add more repetitions in a set.

Wall Squats with Bicep Curls

3 sets of 10–15 repetitions

You will need dumbbells or plastic water bottles. Make sure you use a weight that challenges you without making your muscles hurt (beginner: small dumbbells or small, full water bottles; intermediate/advanced: 3kg dumbbells and above or 750ml–1ltr full water bottles).

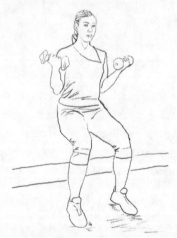

- Start in the position shown.
- Your legs will work isometrically (without movement) by keeping you in position.
- Feet should be at least 30cm (12in) from the wall, pelvis, mid-back and shoulder blades against the wall for support.
- Think of leaning against the wall in a 'good posture' position.

- The only movement to occur is with the arms.
- As you breathe in, ease the dumbbells down beside your legs.
- As you breathe out, pull the dumbbells back up, bending your elbows to the start position.
- To get the most efficient use of the arm muscles keep the elbows tucked in to the sides of your body throughout entire movement.
- Keep your abdominal wall gently tight throughout without pushing your lower back into the wall.
- The back of your head should touch the wall as well – you can do this by pulling the chin back and in, but ensure you feel comfortable.

Double Arm Rows
3 sets of 8–12 repetitions

You can use tins, dumbbells, kettlebells or bags of groceries to help with this one.

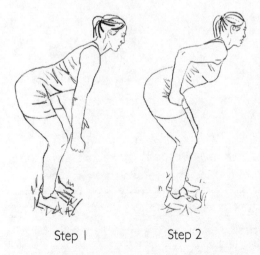

Step 1   Step 2

Both knees should be bent, then bending from the waist, tip over so that your torso is at a 45-degree angle to the floor.

- Engage abdominal and lower back muscles to ensure a safe position and work your core muscles.
- Breathe in, don't move.

- Begin with cans, dumbbells, kettlebells or bags full of groceries below your shoulders (Step 1), arms hanging, then, breathing out, pull both arms up at the same time, bringing the hands to touch the hips, elbows kept in and forearms moving up to a 90-degree angle (Step 2).
- Breathe in to lower the arms to the start position.

Lunges

3 sets of 6–12 on each side

You will need dumbbells, tins or kettlebells.

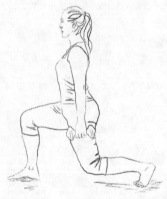

Start by standing with feet together, holding dumbbells, cans or kettlebells in hands.

- Take a long step forward with one foot.
- Keeping your torso in 'good posture', breathe in to ease your way to the position shown here, bending your knees.
- Only go to a position where the knees feel comfortable; you will still achieve a good workout even if you only do a quarter or half of the position shown – the important thing is that you feel safe through all joints.
- Stand up to the start position on an out-breath.
- Complete 6–12 repetitions on one side, then switch to the other leg.
- Keep abdominal muscles gently tight while moving, and torso perpendicular to the floor (upright).

The Bridge (Hamstring and Glute Lifts)
3–6 repetitions held for 10 seconds each

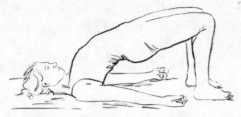

See the instructions on page 215.

Oblique Abdominal Rollback
2 sets of 3 on each side

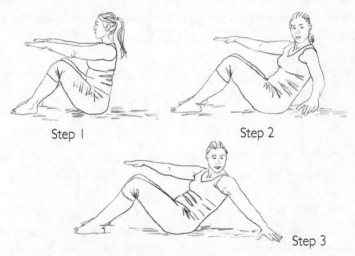

Step 1
Step 2
Step 3

Begin in the seated position (Step 1).

- Breathe in, staying centred.
- Breathe out, drop the sacrum (triangular bum bone) down to the floor as you twist to the left and tighten the abdominal muscles as you imagine pulling the bottom portion of your rib cage towards your hip bones, forming a C-curve through the lower back (Step 2). Think of pulling your belly button and breastbone through your back to create a strong connection.

- Extend your left hand (Step 3), following it with your eyes.
- Breathe in to return to the starting position (Step 1).
- Repeat the movement to the right.
- Shoulder blades (shoulder girdle) stay in a 'good posture' position throughout the movement.
- Movement happens at the pelvis, lower back (flexion) and the shoulder joints.

Cool-down

Don't simply spring up out of these exercises and leave in a flurry of stress. Spend a minute or two stretching your muscles and relaxing. Any of the yoga options in the next chapter, held for a few breaths, will make great post-workout stretches.

If you are pressed for time, the following three exercises will stretch the key muscles you have worked. Hold each stretch for 5–10 relaxed breaths.

1. **Quad/thigh stretch** – Lying on your tummy, bend your right knee and grasp the ankle with your right hand, keeping your pelvis and the rest of your body on the floor – your left hand can be palm-down with your forehead resting on it. Repeat on the other side.

2. **Hip/piriformis stretch** – Stand facing a flight of stairs – bring your right foot onto the second or third step (so, about knee-height), then roll the foot so your little toe and ankle bone are in contact with the step. This bends the knee and opens the hip joint. If you already feel a stretch deep in the hip or bottom area stay standing in this position, holding the hand rail/banister. If you need more of a stretch, lean forward from the hips to support yourself with your hands on the same step or slightly higher. An outdoor option would be to use the back of a bench instead of stairs.

3. **Doorway chest stretch** – Stand in a doorway, bringing both forearms and hands to touch the door frame on their respective sides (arms now stay relaxed). Keep your elbows lower than your shoulders, step through the doorway (leading with your right

foot), bend both knees slightly for support. Lean your shoulders, chest, ribcage and pelvis through the doorway to feel a stretch across the chest and shoulders – keep your shoulders down away from your ears. An outdoor alternative would be at a children's playground with space between poles which is the same width as a doorway (in most playgrounds there will be play structures that have poles).

Spontaneous Activity

A crucial component of De-Stress Fitness is what we call 'spontane-ous' or 'background' activity. This isn't necessarily about putting on your workout clothes and heading off to do structured exercise at the gym twice a week, but about moving around more often and increasing the amount of activity in your day.[9] One of the downsides to the rise of gym culture is that, having worked out in the gym a couple of times a week, people may think being sedentary the rest of the time is okay. It's not – and the sudden shift from 0–100 miles an hour can shock the body and cause the very stress we're trying to avoid. To optimize our metabolisms, we need to move regularly throughout the day – ideally a little every hour.

Some scientists also call this 'incidental' exercise, as it's simply about moving more in the context of your day – wherever you are, whenever you can.[10] Here are some ideas:

Walking

If the De-Stress Diet had a favourite form of exercise, walking would be it. It clears the mind, increases mood and yes, burns calories, but crucially, walking doesn't cost us our energy or stress out the joints and muscles in the way that running can. We evolved to walk or lightly jog. When humans and other primates run, their energy costs are twice those of other mammals. From an energy-balance and stress-reducing perspective, walking is much more efficient. If you take up nothing else from the DSD exercise plan, we urge you to get walking.

Get a pedometer and aim to clock up between 10,000 and 12,500 steps a day about 5 or 6 times a week.[11] Every step counts, even walking to the kitchen to make a tea, but, roughly speaking, 5,000 steps is about half an hour's walking. Studies show that owning a dog encourages sticking to an exercise plan, improves fitness and reduces excess weight. In short, a pooch is not only loyal, it gives you a doe-eyed reason to clock up those steps every day (and a whole load of de-stressing unconditional love).[12] If you're a runner, log on to de-stressyourlife.com for expert tips on ensuring you're not over-stressing your body.

Taking the Stairs

Research published in the *British Journal of Sports Medicine* found that women who ran up and down the stairs at work for 2 minutes at a time, 5 times a day boosted their fitness over an 8-week period.[13] Most of us are time-poor, but if you get up and move around every hour or so by running up a couple of flights of stairs, you're keeping your metabolism more fired up than if you were sitting down for 4 hours straight until lunchtime.

Other Spontaneous Activities

* carrying shopping bags home – evenly distribute the weight over both arms

* having sex (a great de-stressor)

* gardening

* cycling to and from work

* stroller-walking

* vigorous housework

* carrying and chasing after a baby

* doing DIY

* dancing

Fit to Rest

Hunter-gatherers had a practical reason for being fit: so they could feed their families and survive. According to exercise physiologists who study them, hunter-gatherers would have had a widely varied system of movement and would have alternated difficult days with less demanding days whenever they could in order that their cells could be renewed and rebuilt through adequate rest. High-activity days would have been followed by low-activity days.[14,15] This would have reduced the likelihood of crippling injuries and given the body a chance to recharge itself. In fact, while we know that physical exercise has many protective health benefits including lowering our blood pressure and risk of heart disease, there is accumulating evidence showing that extreme physical activities over a prolonged period may be detrimental to health.[16] The pattern of exercise that we are best genetically suited to is a variety of activities performed intermittently and with different levels of intensity – not always high – with adequate rest in between to ensure complete bodily and muscle recovery between exertions.

Marathons, triathlons and very long-distance bike rides don't match the way our bodies evolved to move. According to Charlene's experience, when a seasoned long-distance exerciser or athlete trains over a year-long period, they are periodizing their programme in such a structure that they have short, long, interval and variable training days mixed with rest or active recovery days. But lay people and the 'recreational elite' (those who do the odd triathlon or marathon) are often the ones who get injured or burned out because they train too hard, too soon, believing the training should match the length and intensity of the race. This can exhaust the adrenals, leading to Stressed and Tired.

Alternate

If you do a short strength workout one day, rest your muscles the next. This is crucial. Muscles and connective tissues need time to adapt to the mini-stressors that strength exercise puts on them, and they can't do this without rest. Alternating hard workouts with easy ones and rest days produces better long-term fitness and has a far greater effect on your mood.

Active Relaxation

In Chapter 11 you will learn the simple moving, breathing and meditating techniques that can help your body and muscles to relax. This will allow the action of the parasympathetic nervous system, which is responsible for your recovery from stress. It's crucial to incorporate some relaxation into any fitness routine to counteract the stress that exercise places on the body and to take healthy breathing patterns into the way you move.

Vary It

You may have noticed that this workout programme has different elements. There is no one-size-fits-all form of fitness, and DSD movement is designed to get you active in lots of different ways that suit you, so that exercise becomes a bigger part of your everyday life instead of yet another thing on your to-do list or another reason to feel guilty. Remember that this is what suits your body, not your ambition; check you are listening to how you feel, not think. Don't feel the need to cram all the elements of DSD fitness into any given week. Instead, try and keep variety in mind by opting for the various elements of the programme at the times they fit your life and energy levels.

Active Rest

In his book, *The Power of Rest: why sleep alone is not enough*, US sleep and body-clock researcher Dr Matthew Edlund talks about the types of *active* rest our bodies need. Sleep and watching TV are both types of passive rest, but more essential to rewiring and renewing our bodies are other forms of active rest. As most of us get about seven hours' sleep – a third of us get fewer than five! – other types of rest are essential for deep inner and outer renewal of our minds and bodies. If you're wondering what 'rest' is doing in a chapter on exercise, it's because, for the De-Stress Diet, adequate rest in all its forms is an essential aspect of fitness. So relax, it's compulsory. In the next chapter we outline the yoga and breathing techniques that will help you deeply relax daily, while the box on page 182 outlines signs that you need recovery.

Dr Edlund's Types of Essential Active Rest
Physical Rest
Physical rest is an active, deliberate form of relaxation in which you use your body's basic physical processes such as breathing to calm and restore your body and mind. The deep breathing, restorative yoga and guided relaxation explained in Chapter 11 are these types of rest, as would be a 15-minute (30-minute maximum) daytime nap.

Social Rest
Human beings evolved as social beings, that's why we need to connect with friends we trust and whose company we enjoy to truly recharge and fortify ourselves. A huge bank of studies has shown that the one factor that differentiates happy people from not so happy souls is the power of their connections with others. Social withdrawal is a key sign of low serotonin, Stressed and Demotivated types. Social interaction also releases beta-endorphins and helps break the vicious cycle.

Edlund describes 'social rest' as doing any or all of the following regularly: making a special one-to-one connection with someone you care about, visiting a neighbour or co-worker you would like to get to know better, making quick, useful social connections (think Facebook, Twitter et al.), going for a walk and a chat with a friend in the park. For us, the single greatest – and most de-stressing – example of social rest is laughter. Whether it's a phone call with the person who most makes you laugh, stand-up comedy, rom-coms or bad taste jokes, if you do nothing else as social rest, find something or someone that makes you laugh, and get giggling.

Mental Rest
While in physical rest, you use your body's physical processes to calm and restore. In mental rest, you use your concentration to focus

attention on something beyond your body – this has a deeply restful effect. Examples of mental rest include walking to music, taking garden walks and simple meditation techniques such as mindfulness aware- ness (see Chapter 11). Plus, doing anything where you find time passes quickly – such as a hobby – shows you have reached the meditative 'alpha' brainwave state where we can mentally rejuvenate. You can see therestdoctor.com for more of Dr Edlund's work.[17]

Listen to Your Body

Learn the difference between being simply demotivated and needing to rest:

You need to rest or keep your exercise gentle if you:

- feel heavy and lethargic morning after morning upon waking
- have a feeling of having 'heavy legs' day after day
- when trying a light workout, feel that this strong fatigue or 'heavy legs' still exists
- feel exhausted after exercise.

You're demotivated and might benefit from a workout if you:

- fantasize about lying on the sofa instead of doing something ac- tive or sociable
- feel that working out is 'too hard'
- can come up with detailed excuses to convince yourself that 25 minutes' working out is a bad idea (we have kept your strength workout short to help conserve both energy and time)
- attempt a workout and after about 10 minutes feel a renewed sense of energy – if you don't feel refreshed after exercise, you need more rest.

Flexibility

Many people say 'I can't do yoga because I'm not flexible enough,' shying away from it because the initial releasing and lengthening of muscle can feel intense. In Chapter 11 we discuss the attitudes and perceptions you need to do this intelligently, but be assured, just like movement, your body is designed for flexibility to continually open all of your connective tissue.

What Is Flexibility?

The mobility and agility of your body depends on the strength and ability of the connective tissues around your joints to expand and contract freely. Age, a sedentary lifestyle and even too much over-exercise and repetitive movement can mean muscles contract around joints and this can limit our range of movement, leading to some of the aches and pains we associate with old age. But this isn't necessarily inevitable. By treating flexibility and stretching as essential and important parts of your De-Stress Diet movement programme, you could help prevent the loss of mobility that many experience as they get older. Anything from 10–90 minutes a day stretching, in the form of yoga, Pilates or dance stretching, alongside the posture and breathing considerations discussed in the next chapter, will benefit your body and mind in the following ways:

Fewer Injuries

By lengthening the connective tissues, muscles and ligaments between the joints, the body's range of movement is expanded – and this can reduce the likelihood and severity of injuries both from exercise and everyday life.[18]

Improved Posture and Muscle Appearance

Flexibility training slowly lengthens muscles and decreases muscle 'bulk' without sacrificing healthy, lean tissue. It also strengthens the core muscles, which can make the body appear leaner, longer and more toned.[19]

Delays the Onset of Tired Muscles

Stretching adequately after exercise can also help muscles recover more quickly and prevent post-workout muscle soreness.[20]

Mind and Body Become Comfortable with 'Good Pain'

That point where a muscle stretch feels challenging but you can still relax is a good form of stress on the body. It's the point at which you take a stretch to its safe and comfortable limit without any tension in other areas of the body to compensate.

Helps Promote a Feeling of Deep Mental Wellbeing

By urging muscles to relax, and promoting the stretching of key nerves that link the joints to the mind, flexibility training can have profoundly De-Stressing benefits in as little as 15 minutes.[21] Our preferred form of flexibility training is yoga because of its emphasis on breath and stilling the mind (see the following chapter).

Get Together

Studies have shown that people get a boost in mood when they have the chance to socialize with friends, family and colleagues.[22] Ironically, those of us who are more introverted may benefit most from such interaction. 'Social Setting Exercise' – that is, any activity that requires more than one person to perform – is an essential part of DSD fitness not only for its cardiovascular effects but also for its ability to help you connect with other people, have fun and engage in some healthy competition. We are pack animals and cohesion of the tribe is key to survival, so our brains reward these behaviours with a shot of the happy chemical dopamine. These are all multi-beneficial forms of De-Stressing that get us out of our over-stimulated mental states and help us burn off the stress hormones generated during a typical working week.

Engage in Social Setting Exercise 1–2 times a week. This could be anything you enjoy that requires more than one person. It can be done after work or at weekends to incorporate family and social gatherings. Pleasurable activities can provide a boost in wellbeing, and in studies looking at activities that increase positive mood, those that caused the greatest benefits for people were those they enjoyed the most.

Our favourite Social Setting Exercise forms incorporate proven emotional as well as physical wellbeing benefits, raising feel-good beta-endorphins and the anti-stress hormone DHEA:

- **Dancing** For hunter-gatherers, dancing would have been performed as part of rituals and cultural celebrations and would have burned a massive 500 calories an hour. More importantly, we also know dancing not only improves fitness, it also reduces stress. In fact, it's also been shown to improve memory, mood and cognitive (brain) functioning in the elderly and to help lower blood pressure.[23]

- **Having sex** Large studies have found that people who have sex regularly report a host of health benefits including raised immune function and lower mortality and risk of heart disease. A vigorous session of active sex can burn up to 200 calories. It's often the last thing we feel like doing when we're stressed, but when we make ourselves get started, it's not long before we're enjoying ourselves, right? In fact, even a 'quickie' can make us feel better. That's because sex works towards our wellbeing on a chemical as well as physical level. It stimulates our bodies to produce hormones called prolactin and oxytocin, which are associated with improvements in mood and psychological bonding.[24,25]

- **Nature hikes** We mentioned above the extensive studies showing the psychological as well as physical benefits of exercising outdoors. Add the challenging and often strenuous yet beautiful terrain you're negotiating on hikes and you have a winning example of the perfect De-Stress Social Setting Exercise. A study in 2008 of groups hiking along the Appalachian Trail in the US reported multiple benefits including physical challenge, self-fulfilment, warm relationships with others, fun, enjoyment of life and of course, great exercise.[26]

Negative Ions: Positive Vibes from Outdoor Exercise

Some researchers believe that the reason we feel so good at the seaside, in a rainforest or near a running waterfall is because the air in such natural places is charged with negative ions. These are taste-less, odourless and invisible molecules in certain environments such as mountains, beaches and forests believed to produce biochemical reactions that increase levels of the mood-chemical serotonin, helping to alleviate depression, relieve stress and increase energy. Conversely, it's also believed that one of the reasons we can feel more stressed in cities, air-conditioned buildings or more polluted areas is that the air in such environments is said to be charged with *positive* ions which might increase stress, tension and tiredness (computer monitors also emit positive ions).[27]

Here are some more suggestions for Social Setting exercise:

- tennis
- badminton
- rowing
- squash
- Green Gym – This is the local clearing and gardening of green public spaces run by the charity BCTV throughout the UK in group settings. A warning: it's strenuous but excellent fun.
- outdoor swimming

In the tools section at de-stressyourlife.com you will find the addresses and websites for some societies and clubs in Britain that will get you started.

Get Outside

Vitamin D deficiency is becoming an epidemic in people who work long hours and see little light, and research is now showing that ad-equate levels are essential to both mood and weight management, as well as bone health and cancer prevention.[28] The best source for humans is UV light on the skin.[29] If you can't get outside to work out, spend 10 minutes outside in direct sunlight exposing your face and forearms, or 30 minutes when it is dull or cloudy, without sunscreen every day to boost your Vitamin D levels.

At the University of Essex, researchers have extensively studied the wellbeing effects of outdoor exercise and have found that three-quarters of outdoor exercisers tested felt less angry, depressed or tense, compared with only half who worked out in a gym. Plus, the same team has also found that only 5 minutes in nature can have a positive impact on mood.[30] We have a synergy with green plants: they oxygenate us while using our waste gas carbon dioxide for their own energy production. We breathe more deeply in the countryside, whereas in the face of pollution we protect ourselves with more shallow breathing.

Exercise outdoors whenever you can, even if it means starting out cold. One study found that women who walked outside experienced more elevations in mood after their walks than those who walked inside.[31] Being outside in the fresh air also increases the thermogenic effects of exercise. The more you recondition yourself to live in slightly colder conditions, the more you reset your body to burn fat rather than store it.

Exercising outside while being exposed to natural light has also been shown to help alleviate the symptoms of depression.[32] Spending time outside exposed to natural light helps balance hormones such as melatonin and cortisol that govern your body's sleep/wake cycle. It also helps prevent the onset of Seasonal Affective Disorder that causes seasonal depression in the winter.

LabChat: Cool Down

Remember thermogenics from Chapter 1, which can help sneakily burn fat by forcing the body to raise its own temperature. Two simple ways to do this are to lower the thermostat at home to below 22 degrees Celsius and to turn on the cold tap for 30 seconds at the end of your shower each morning. A study in the New England Journal of Medicine found making yourself cold activates 'brown fat', a healthy type of fat in the body that increases metabolism and burns off 'white fat', the less active kind[33]. Brown fat is present in babies and we lose it as we get older but researchers have found that adults can help reactivate theirs by lowering their temperatures.

Help for Your Specific Stress Suit

All types can benefit from the resistance training above and the yoga, breathing and relaxation techniques outlined in Chapter 11, with these specific exercise considerations taken into account:

	Best Exercise by Stress Suit
Stressed and Wired	Slow down, especially if you have become addicted to the hard workout. Recovery is crucial as you learn to relax. If you're a jogger, do walk/jog sessions with light jogging to lessen the risk of overtraining; in this way you can achieve the feeling of a hard workout without the stress hormones. Also try walking, Pilates and easy swimming. Stay away from any hard cardiovascular activities. Choose activities low on competition to relieve the stressful need to achieve.
Stressed and Tired/ Stressed and Cold	Choose outdoor walks/activities for fresh air, with time to breathe and come out of 'daytime fog'. Schedule workouts/activities during the day if possible so that energy has had time to build up. Don't force evening workouts as these can tire you out even more.
Stressed and Bloated	Avoid activities lying on your tummy as this can feel uncomfortable. Try Pilates or yoga poses which are in seated or standing positions with neutral back instead of lying on a mat. Outdoor walks or activities in the fresh air increase abdominal circulation. Leave 2–3 hours after eating before exercising.

Stressed and Sore	If you have joint pain, avoid impact activities with bouncing, jumping or landing. Weight training is a must to strengthen bones and maintain healthy joint lubrication. Avoid long, hard cardiovascular workouts and choose walk/jogs or walking instead. If hay fever or asthma is triggered by pollen, switch to indoors at these times of year. Watch stress levels closely to avoid setting off inflammatory responses. Hydrate well so inflammatory histamines are less likely to be produced in the body after exercise.
Stressed and Demotivated	Opt for group classes for socialization such as aquarobics, dancing and other low-intensity classes. Substitute late-night binges for meditation, restorative yoga or walking. Morning workouts can help to increase feelings of vitality and mood, especially in the winter months. Buddy/friend workouts help motivate you to attend and add a social aspect proven to lift mood.
Stressed and Hormonal	Opt for group classes for support and socialization. Move every day – exercise is crucial for hormone balance through circulation and detoxification. Yoga and meditation help with irritability, crying and negative thoughts. Walking at times of your period or sugar cravings can aid in decreasing pain and take your mind off cravings.

Chapter 11
CALM FOR LIFE

The breath awareness and mindfulness within yoga practice are, along with natural movement and nutrition, key tools used in The De-Stress Diet to help you find slim and calm. Once you have explored and practised the techniques in this chapter, you will return to them again and again to help you find balance, relaxation and space in everyday life, and to turn to in your most stressful moments. Like everything in this book, they are designed to be practical and accessible. More than anything else, the techniques here are designed to help you find moments of stillness within your life.

Yoga, Breathing, Mindfulness

- Yoga asanas (postures/poses) help prepare body and mind for meditation, and have the added beneficial side-effects of improved posture, strength and flexibility. They are positions that we wouldn't usually place our bones, muscles and joints in during everyday life, which presents a 'good stress' challenge for us physically, evoking a positive response from circulation, muscle strength, release and length, hormonal balance and oxygenation through breath – but only when we are breathing easily and with focused awareness.

- Yoga poses open your body to counter the effects of stress, such as muscles tightened by the fight-or-flight response, postural shut-down from sitting on chairs and lack of continual natural movement.

- The easy breathing techniques and practices in this chapter will help you cope with stress and bring you into the calming parasympathetic state when life feels claustrophobic or overwhelming.

- Finding mindfulness needn't take the shape of formalized meditation, but can be used in any activity such as washing up, gardening, walking – wherever you can be fully focused and present. Practising mindfulness when you eat will help you chew and fully digest, and increase appetite regulation by sending the right signals back to your brain.

- Learning to stay with yoga postures, breathing practices and meditation helps us to become more accepting and able to relax into what might previously have been perceived as discomfort or pain. What are simply strong sensations of release during a stretch or change on a bigger scale can cause us to react with sudden contractions or aversions. Conditioning ourselves to breathe and relax in the face of these strong sensations helps us acclimatize to good, natural physical stress – these include exercise, intellectual challenges, being a little cold, even feeling true hunger – and become stronger. In fact, 15,000 long-term yoga practitioners were assessed by researchers and shown to put on lower-than-average weight over 10 years. The study does not draw conclusions, but one theory is that this is because yoga practice makes us more able to resist the discomfort of cravings.[1]

Breath Awareness

Practising the postures or any other aspect of yoga without looking for connection with your breath and body is simply making shapes. A stretch is just a stretch if you are not fully engaged with the process of opening that this brings. Even if you choose not to make the yoga posture sequences in this chapter part of your De-Stress routine, breathing awareness and mindfulness will make a huge difference to the way you deal with the stress in your everyday life.

Breathing is the clearest signal of your body's state at any given time. Pulling air into the body and then releasing the waste product carbon dioxide involves large sets of muscles and can differ depending on the state of your body and mind as well as what is going on around you. We can see different states affecting the breath:

1. Diaphragmatic breathing – This uses the primary breathing muscles, the large upside-down-bowl-shaped diaphragm muscles at the bottom of your ribs, with an easy exchange of filling and emptying the lungs, chest expanding to inhale and diaphragm rising back up to exhale. When you're lying down this breathing can be seen as the belly rising and falling. It is the most energy-efficient, oxygenating breath and least stressful to the muscular system.

2. Thoracic (chest) breathing – When we're stressed or if there is not enough room for the diaphragm to move fully, breath moves to the upper chest and shoulders. During the fight-or-flight response, this causes quicker, shallow breaths. Many people get stuck in this pattern, using up precious energy and creating tension in the neck and upper back.[2]

The Nasal Breath

When stressed, many of us breathe through our mouth rather than nose, which is particularly problematic on the in-breath. Mouth-breathing is associated with the poor posture and lack of oxygenation that cause tiredness.[3] In yoga, all breathing unless otherwise instructed is through the nose. Nasal breathing cools down the frontal lobe of the brain, which calms its activity and warms up air entering the lungs and body for easy oxygen uptake. It also helps the body produce nitric oxide, which is important for immune function and circulation. Yogis maintain that *prana* (life-force) from the breath is only taken into the body through the nose (as well as through food and sunlight). If you have nasal issues that make this difficult, look at the immune and inflammatory advice in the Stressed and Sore section on pages 34–35 to reduce mucus. Reducing stress and improving posture can help you to change breathing patterns safely and organically.

The Best De-Stress Tool

Breathing is part of the autonomic nervous system. It happens automatically and changes continually. But by becoming aware of how we breathe, we are able consciously to change this and stop the vicious cycles of chronic breathing issues signalling back to the nervous system that we are in danger. In yoga, calm, long breaths increase oxygenation, spare vital nutrients, reduce heart rate, relax muscles and reduce anxiety. This increases all-over communication throughout the body, including that between the brain, spinal cord and nerves. Therefore, it quiets the mind. The brain needs three times more oxygen than the rest of the body; so increasing this supply with conscious breathing can have immediate positive effects on mood, cognitive function and focus.

Breathing awareness in yoga is called *pranayama*, and though often practised as specific types of breathing, it also refers to all conscious breathing. For a stressed nervous system, controlling the breath into specific counts or patterns can actually create more stress. A research study on stress management showed that, for 15 people with daily tension and 13 with panic disorder, paying attention to the breath slowed breathing down, whereas specific breathing instructions showed no relaxation of tendencies to breathe quickly.[4]

Many yoga students are instructed that the ideal breath length ratio is 1:2 inhalation to exhalation, but if your natural rhythm differs in any way or the day's events have thrown you off-track, pushing a round peg into a square hole is not the solution. Stepping back from yet more control in our lives and simply letting the breath be in its calmest, fullest and most natural state is more conducive to connecting to what we need. This is the basis for our breathing recommendations.

First, let's look at what is happening during a single breath:

- Inhalation – pulling the air into the body involves muscular contraction and creates energy, but can bring in more tension if it's done with force. Better to fully exhale, creating a vacuum into which the in-breath can flow effortlessly. The most efficient and easy inhalation comes with posture that has least tension.

- Exhalation – at its best, this is simply letting go of the muscles that pulled in the in-breath. Stress can tend to make you breathe in over the end of the out-breath, so focusing on allowing the exhalation to drift right to its natural end-point helps its calming parasympathetic action. The exhalation can start to become naturally longer as shoulders, chest and jaw relax more.

The First Sign You're Stressed

You may not normally notice, but when you are stressed the first thing to change is your breathing. Begin looking out for signs of stress in your breath – this is the time when even the shortest breathing break can make all the difference:

- Hyperventilation – or over-breathing. This is the rapid breath where more oxygen than the body needs is taken in the face of panic or stress and can be accompanied by numbness, dizziness, headache and nervous laughter.

- Yawning – new research shows that yawning is the body's way of cooling the brain, a signal that you could benefit from a breathing break during cerebral tasks and stressful times.[5]

- Sighing – this acts like a reset button for breathing that has become out of whack by loosening the air sacs that can get tightened by stressed breathing.[6] If you catch yourself sighing often, you may be a breath-holder: this is your body's way of making up an oxygen deficit.

- Breath-holding – this is a habit we can learn in childhood that sticks; we can be unaware that we have learned to hold our breath in the face of fear, excitement, even joy but it creates adrenaline to make us more focused. Yoga breathing practices that call for retaining the breath should be practised only with caution and expert instruction if any stress is present.

10 Deep Breaths

Before you eat and whenever you feel tension rising, breath quickening or holding, inhalation dominating, tightness around the skull or panic, stop, sit if possible and create a De-Stress breathing-space:

- If around people, simply take several deep, full, natural inhalations to signal a series of however many full, spacious exhalations you need to release, feeling your face and jaw relax.

- If alone, take a deep nasal inhalation, as if you are smelling something lovely like a rose. Breathe out through your mouth, fully opening and sighing out with any natural noise if appropriate. Open your jaw and stick out your tongue with the out breath if you feel it helps release stress deep into your jaw and skull. Swallow if you need to help release throat tension.

- Just 5–10 of these breaths can calm you down and bring you into the present, helping to minimize panic or impulsive stress-related reactions.

The more you get used to practising this tool in the face of stress, the more your body will automatically use this technique with less conscious thought from you. You can also use it to prevent force from entering your yoga poses and to help you find the intuitive length of a pose.

Longer Breathing Practices

We encourage you to take time out, even just a few minutes daily for conscious breathing practice. Conscious breathing can prepare you to cope with the stresses of the coming day, or help you let go of them at the end. Every little helps: one minute achieved is better than planning 20 minutes and then doing nothing but creating the pointless stress of failure. Here's how:

1. Get Comfortable

Although most images of breathing exercises are in a sitting position, this is only recommended if you feel absolutely no tension in the neck, shoulders, chest, back or hips. It is better to be fully supported in a way that allows the whole body to rest and the chest to open easily. In no way should you feel slumped or stressed, or as if you are swimming upstream rather than going with the tide:

- Lying in Savasana (page 221) or better, in the lift shown in Supta Baddha Konasana (page 220) with legs out straight allows full diaphragmatic breathing as the chest is fully supported.

- Definitely don't sit if you tend to nod off while in Savasana. This is a sign you are overtired, and sitting would stress you further. If you sleep there, you probably need to – go with it (it took Charlotte years to stay awake in restorative poses!).

- Sitting on a chair is an option if tightness in the hips makes chest-opening tense. Support the lower back with a cushion for ease sitting upright.

- You may feel that sitting in Siddhasana (page 209) is comfortable for you, but practise poses that loosen the shoulders and hips and open the chest first.

2. Relax

The simplest practice is also to be observed in all breathing, yoga and even daily life: that your face stays soft. Frowning sends a message to the brain that you must be tense, while a soft jaw and face – even a little smile – tells the body that things must be okay and you can relax. Every so often, check that:

- You are not clenching your jaw or gritting your teeth, even opening the jaw wide to release around the ear socket and the base of the skull.

- You are soft across the forehead, around the temples and between the eyebrows.

- You release tension upwards from the lower body; held in hips, lower back, belly, groin, chest, upper spine and shoulders. This tension can get 'stuck' in the upper chest, throat and jaw. Do the above and swallow where needed, releasing shoulders away from the ears.

3. Choose a Breathing Tool

Choose one of the following tools and begin to observe your breath flow in and out as naturally as possible. Watch your nervous system calm down, relaxing the brain, muscles and whole body. Cultivate this sense of safety and self-protection. The more you consciously do this, the more your body and mind can always find a safe, energizing, calming place.

- Simply observe your breath like a tide, naturally flowing in and out with no expectation or imposition, right to the end. Use any rhythmic soothing imagery that resonates with you, seeing the breath as a swing, hammock, wave, leaf on the wind…

- Watch the inhalation rise up from the end of your tailbone to the crown of your head, and then observe the exhalation release back down all the way to the end of your spine.

- Say the internal mantra 'Let' on the inhalation, 'Go' on the exhalation to give the instruction 'Let go' to your whole body. This is often a useful intervention if you are really tense.

- Focus on releasing each out-breath further and further away from your head, so that you move away from any thoughts and become more connected to your root around the belly and pelvic floor, where you feel rather than think. It may help you to imagine this area as red energy if that comes easily.

- Focus on your heart centre (which you may easily visualize as nourishing green energy if this happens naturally), breathing in to feel compassion and unconditional loving kindness to yourself. This is particularly helpful if you tend to give out lots of energy to others at the expense of yourself.

- Visualize the exhalation making space by releasing stagnant energy, tension and anything that doesn't serve you; then the inhalation comes in naturally to fill the space with fresh, new energy and oxygen which you see filling every part of your body.

- This simple variation of the Buddhist meditation 'Mindfulness of Breathing' helps train awareness of the breath: Begin counting '1' on the inhalation, '1' on the exhalation. Continue counting the full breath cycle like this up to 10, then start again. If your mind wanders or you lose count, simply start again at 1.

Mindfulness Meditation

Images of yogis and monks sitting for hours can put a huge barrier of expectation between you and accessing this profound but simple state. We all enter altered states of consciousness throughout the day. It is our brain's way of switching off momentarily to regroup and have a little power rest. If you've ever suddenly realized you've been staring off into space for minutes without noticing, that's your body taking its own little meditation break. Meditation means concentrating and focusing on this state, to allow your mind and body to be consciously in the present moment without attaching to thoughts that pull you away. But it doesn't have to be done cross-legged with candles and gongs. Mindfulness meditation can be done anywhere and is about bringing focus to whatever you are doing to truly experience it and be in the present.

Mindfulness Anywhere

Our hope here is to give you permission to find meditation and mindfulness however and wherever suits you. You can meditate formally (see breathing positions above and meditation tips on page 199) or practise mindfulness while doing a simple repetitive activity such as ironing, gardening or stuffing envelopes if you cut out background stimulus (from TVs, radios, etc.). You can actively watch your breath, shoulders and jaw release, and find natural relaxation when you create the space to allow this to happen. Many people find activities such as swimming or walking meditative, and as ways of optimizing the free time you have to both move and relax the brain. This is why Charlotte always urges clients to just walk in nature whenever possible, with no iPod or phone calls to distract or stimulate them. Mindfulness means cultivating awareness of the present and being there, rather than being away in thoughts of the past or future. Sitting on a park bench for 1 or 2 minutes is a vast improvement on never finding any time for centring yourself.

It is this state of mindfulness that we should use while eating, and is how our digestive and appetite regulation mechanisms are set to work optimally. Being mindful and present while you eat involves sitting and simply eating, being aware of chewing, tasting and savouring every single mouthful – not working, walking to the tube, reading, watching TV, surfing the net or walking round the house on the phone. We have become addicted to distraction, the essence of mindlessness, and that's how we end up ploughing in food we haven't even noticed we've eaten.

Meditation

Meditation is part of every true yoga practice; it is the absorption, focus and concentration we are moving towards when we practise the postures. It can take a formal form in a sequence, or create an attitude within which to integrate body and mind intelligently, keeping us aware of when we might allow habits like force, ego or ambition to enter our practice. For example, in a pose such as Cat/Cow (page 210), the rhythmic movement of the spine can become a 'moving meditation' where we fully let the breath rather than the brain lead the movement.

Don't Force Emptying the Mind

A common subtle misconception about meditation is that it is about 'emptying the mind', provoking actions of pushing away thoughts. This can be a forceful act in a busy brain, so instead of wrestling with your 'chattering monkeys', use the following tools as you practise your meditation and mindfulness activities:

1. Cultivate non-reaction. The basis of meditation is not pushing away thoughts but acknowledging them without getting involved. This helps us to simply step to one side, become the observer and cultivate non-attachment, not letting individual thoughts become larger stories in our minds.

2. Always let the out-breath guide you back down from the brain to occupy your whole body.

3. Watch tendencies for self-doubt, anger, resentment, restlessness and boredom to steal you away from focusing on the breath. These tendencies are natural; in the words of Swami J (<u>swamij. com</u>), 'Let them all come and let them all go'.

4. This is both simple and complicated. Don't judge your practice, it is what it is and it will always differ. Whether your meditation feels easy or difficult, makes you feel happy, angry or sad, it will always benefit you.[7,8,9]

Yoga

Many people – including athletes – start yoga because it really does bring muscular strength, tone, flexibility and endurance to the body. However, most people *continue* it because of the sense of connection, relaxation and contentment it brings to the mind. If you don't already know this through regular yoga practice, you soon will. People who show the same signs of stressful living – including tight breathing, bodies and faces as well as difficulties 'letting go' – respond to conscious breathing and yoga practice with great relief and steady progress, however challenging this can seem in the beginning.

The word *yoga* comes from the Sanskrit word for 'yolk', and translates as 'union'. The original meaning of yoga for the ancient sages who first described this philosophy wasn't about being flexible or acrobatic, but meditating towards a truly reflective state. The postures were added later to help the right breath and energy movement for meditation. We can't over-state this: yoga has become known as a toning tool for the body, but its true emphasis is for the mind and spirit. If you immediately feel a tingle of wariness about the spiritual aspect, ask a few long-term yoga practitioners what this word means to them and you'll find vastly different answers. For Charlotte, yoga means 'Being connected to nature and the world around me, the opposite of being shut down and isolated'. For Anna, yoga translates simply to 'Coming home to my mind and body'.

Yoga's ultimate aim is to attain *Samadhi* – ultimate connection with the universe, a melding of your individual consciousness with the larger world around you. In practical terms this simply means cultivating connection between your breath, body and mind, helping you to find stillness and connect with how you truly feel rather than how you *think* you feel.

This is the basis for focus, intuition and mindfulness within the De-Stress lifestyle – helping you stay with that reflective rather than impulsive self.

The Benefits of Yoga

Some people think of yoga as 'the soft option' – rooms full of people sitting cross-legged. In fact, it's a complete mind and body system that has been practised for over 4,000 years. Scientific studies have revealed the following benefits:

- Reductions in Body Mass Index (BMI), blood pressure and heart rate.[10]

- Increased relaxing alpha brain waves and decreased levels of the stress hormone cortisol; just one hour a week can help reduce stress and anxiety.[11,12]

- Continued, regular practice leads to weight loss, specifically lowered waist-to-hip circumference and body fat levels, better appetite control and postural stability.[13]

- Yoga can also help alleviate headaches, insomnia, sleep issues, depression and lower back pain.[14]

- Two classes a week can help improve menstrual problems as well as food cravings and body image.[15,16]

Yoga for Stress Relief

- All twists massage the adrenal glands and organs to encourage circulation, energy and help you cope with stress.

- Forward bends help to still a racing mind after a busy day.

- Hip- and chest-openers release the back after hunching over a computer.

- Down-face Dog is always safe to bridge or 'neutralize the spine' between any poses, helping prevent injury in a tight body.

- Inversions turn our world upside-down and give our hearts a rest from pumping blood up from the legs. Add a restorative element as in Viparita Karani (page 221) and we can help relieve tired or achy legs, a common symptom of chronic stress.

More details at de-stressyourlife.com

Allowing, Not Pushing

We hold stress in our bodies and can feel physical, emotional and psychological effects as we release areas like the hips and back. To begin with, it's natural to resist and contract around intense feelings, for example during a stretch, labelling them as 'pain'. On stretching a muscle, it will contract first to protect itself while working out if it is safe to lengthen without damage. Easy breathing and a calm nervous system signal this safe release, but this can take up to several minutes for some muscles — you can build more pain and tension if you grit your teeth and push. You make more progress by waiting and *allowing*. This needs full concentration on the area of tension, but also a sense of breathing space around it to facilitate 'letting go' — in Sanskrit this is called *Stira Sukha* or 'focus/steadiness with ease'.

Studies have shown that pain, and our reaction to it, decrease with practice. Massage and yoga have been shown to elicit similar cortisol-lowering effects, with yoga described as 'self-massage' as the limbs rub against each other and the floor. This and increased serotonin levels are believed to help shut down 'pain gateways' in those for whom pain in joints and muscles often prevents exercise.[17]

In life and yoga, we are often drawn to activities that reinforce habits rather than provide what we need. In yoga these habits are called *samskaras*, and it is widely recognized that those who tend to be overstimulated gravitate towards a more dynamic practice when they may need more quiet and calm. Those feeling tired and lethargic can fall into a purely restorative practice, when what they might need are poses that gradually create more energy.[18]

Postural Intelligence

Postural issues are highly individual, but we are all based around the same skeletal structural design. This means that even though we can't assess you or cover every eventuality or solution, we have chosen poses in sequences that help your body best find its own positioning. For those who have engaged in long-term yoga practice, remember that we are never 'finished' with postural work and that it can be like driving: the longer you do it, the more likelihood you can get complacent. In place of being truly attentive to bad habits, you can lose the basics. Continual assessment by an anatomically knowledgeable teacher is important. For those of you with a naturally very flexible body, be careful not to go to the extremes of poses without paying attention. It is better to hold off and strengthen the muscles that hold the pose and create support, rather than pulling on joints and tendons to strive for the 'advanced' posture.

For every posture, observe the following instructions. These are also useful in everyday life as you sit at a desk, drive, walk or take the bus:

1. Make space in your spine – elongating front and back to prevent compression between discs so you can bend and twist safely and freely in all directions.

2. Release your shoulders away from your ears – cultivating diaphragmatic breathing means you don't need to involve the

shoulders in breathing, can lengthen your neck and spine and move your shoulder blades down your back and in towards your ribcage to be able to lift your chest.

3. Support your lower back – engage your abdominal muscles and pelvic floor gently but firmly, and lengthen your tailbone. This can help draw in a 'banana back' and a tendency to stick your bum out. If you tend to cave in at the belly, be careful that these contractions don't worsen this (e.g. curve your back more in Down-face Dog) and draw in and up from the back of your pelvis and breastbone.

4. Draw in your bottom ribs – lifting the breastbone away from the pubic bone can often make us jut out the ribs and feel we are tall when we are actually rather pigeon-chested. Pulling the ribcage back into line helps broaden both across the collarbones and the upper back, avoiding over-bending the lower back.

5. Avoid lifting your chin too much – sitting at computer screens can tend to round the upper back, meaning we have to look up to look forward (sometimes called 'writer's' or 'turtle' neck). Add this to a feeling that lifting the chin means we are proud and motivated and this is a highly common trait. Feel the back and sides of the neck are lengthened to avoid pain and tightness in the neck and upper back. Feel the base of the skull lifting.

6. Soften the jaw – postural tightness follows down the body.

Home Practice

Yoga classes provide the anatomical and instructional attention crucial to safe practice, and we recommend that you find a teacher – if not for weekly classes, then even a few personal sessions or regular workshops. Videos can offer real instruction but cannot give you personal adjustment or advice. Home practice ultimately means the chance to be more intuitive and respond to what you need, but is well supported by classes.

Yoga Classes

1. Find the class that is right for you – beginners' courses can offer a good grounding and give you the space to explore safely without feeling competitive with the bendy person next to you.

2. If you have knee, back, neck or other body issues that concern you, call and talk to the teacher first to be confident he or she has the anatomical knowledge to support you safely and give you options (like props) to practise without creating tension or force. You may also find a dedicated teacher specializing in remedial classes in your area. You need to feel safe and supported in class.

3. Check that your teacher is trained with a school accredited by the Yoga Alliance or British Wheel of Yoga.

4. Try different classes and styles – this keeps your mind open and allows you to see which facilitate you feeling energized, but also calm and not hyped up.

During Your 6-Week Plan

Phase 1: Transition

You begin to learn your natural rhythm and listen to it, but may have periods of discomfort because you're avoiding food and habits that have stressed you in the past. When feeling intense cravings or emotional stress, find the activity or active relaxation from this chapter that helps you stay present. Whether that is yoga asana practice, focused breathing, walking or talking to a supportive friend, be mindful that this is not avoidance but facing being aware of the feelings that are coming up and letting them go, so you can move on. This can include possible panic or anxiety when spending time 'not doing'.

Including yoga in your De-Stress 6-Week Plan and beyond can lead to:

- Decreased binge-eating and eating disorder symptoms.[19]

- Less overeating, more time taken to eat and better food choices.[20]

- A rise in GABA levels (our natural anti-anxiety brain chemical).[21] As GABA can be first lowered when giving up things to which you are addicted, yoga can help you cope with giving up sugar and refined carbohydrates at this time.

Phase 2: True Change

This is where you start to find your natural rhythm and feel more connected and trusting of your instincts. Your appetite should have regulated and your cravings subsided so you begin to experience real hunger and feel more connected to your body. In this phase we urge you to continue practising the sequences and attending a class if you have found one. Long-term yoga practice has been shown to reduce the inflammatory markers associated with stress, and to lead to lower levels of cytokine interleukin-6 (IL-6) which is linked to diabetes, heart disease, stroke, arthritis and other age-related diseases. In short, long-term yoga practice helps you and your body cope well with stress.[22]

The De-Stress Yoga Sequences

Each pose has a simple description to which you can apply the following considerations to experience deeper awareness:

- **Revisit** the 'Postural' (page 203) and 'Breath Awareness' (page 191) sections regularly, to help you carry these into all poses.

- **Entering:** Coming into a pose is as much a part of it as the end picture you see. This also helps set the attitude that, every time you do a pose, it is like the first, different to any other time and treated as such to avoid just 'going through the motions'.

- **Attitude within the pose:** A sense of continual play, exploration and rhythm with the breath keeps poses alive and stops you expecting always to feel the same way. On some days everything will feel right, while on others you may feel resistance and distraction. It is what it is – yoga helps set up an adaptable mind that deals with stress more easily in this way.

- **Time in the pose:** Feel the length of the pose that is right for you at that time, connecting with your intuition rather than a specific breath count. Stay as long as you are able to keep the face, jaw and breath smooth.

- **Leaving:** As with Entering, a graceful departure helps retain the space made. Do not suddenly 'ping' out of a pose because you've been gritting your teeth throughout. This helps smooth transitions between all poses.

- **Side Two:** If you're doing an asymmetrical pose that needs repeating on the other side, approach 'side two' as a whole new pose, not taking assumptions or expectations with you. Start again as mindfully as on side one, so as not to elicit the comparisons that take you back into that analytical brain.

- **Always** come back to this simple phrase to be your guide: 'The breath leads, the body follows and the mind observes'.

More lengthy descriptions, benefits, pose variations, help for different postural needs and more sequences are at de-stressyourlife.com
Check with your doctor before starting any new movement regimen, especially if you have any neck, head, shoulder, arm, wrist, back or knee issues or a tendency to headaches, dizziness, numbness, tingling or high blood pressure. We suggest you read all pose descriptions first to get a feel for the practice with less stress-producing confusion, and then enjoy!

Morning Practice

We have kept this short to provide a tool and attitude to set you up for the day, without creating any sense of pressure that you can't find the time, or feelings of failure if you don't manage it. If morning energy is an issue, a few well-chosen postures, such as those following, cover our full range of motion – standing, back bend, forward bend, twist and hip opening – can help energize the body if you focus on breath and alignment.

We can feel naturally tight in the morning, so work with some energy to spare and space for muscles to wake up gradually. We have extra poses and variety to add at de-stressyourlife.com should you have more time, and recommend that you prioritize the following sequence to prepare your body, mind and nervous system for the day's stresses ahead. Aim for doing this at least 3–4 times a week.

We have highlighted *De-Stress Morning Priority** poses for an even shorter sequence on those difficult days, or as you ease in to a new morning routine. Set an alarm if time pressures introduce stress that steals from your absorption; most phones now have a gong-type ring, rather than something jangly and jarring. Set the ring for 1–2 minutes before you need to stop so you can lie in *Savasana* or sit for this time at least to gather and settle the energy created from the movement.

Don't worry if you haven't completed the sequence fully in the allotted time; this is a good sign that you were moving fully inside the poses and reaching the state of focused exploration that brings most benefit.

If you are finding that this morning practice takes you less time, slow down. This is a sequence designed for you to spend time opening up with *passive* but deeply strengthening stretching that helps lengthen muscles safely. Faster, repetitive motions create *dynamic* stretching, which tends to contract and stress muscles and tendons more. Wanting to rush through can also be a sign that you might tend to be focusing on the broader strokes and the end-point, rather than the smaller subtle aspects of the journey. If you are used to a more vigorous practice, try this different approach with an open mind and maybe to complement other types of practice.

This 16-pose sequence is designed so you can move smoothly between poses. Again, you can focus on the 7 asterisked (*) poses for a shorter sequence.

Siddhasana – Adept's Pose – Loose version*

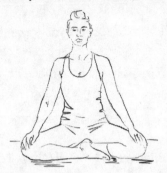

- Sitting on at least one block or cushion to allow lifting from the front spine, take each buttock out and back to sit up from the front of the sitting bones, hands softly on thighs, elbows loose.
- Open the heart from inside the ribcage and lift up to the crown of the head from the back of the skull with each in-breath.
- Open the hips, allowing the legs to drop down with each out-breath. Abdominal support protects and lifts the lower back.
- Release any gripping with the shoulders or knees with the out-breath, as the in-breath lifts the spine.

Parivrtta Siddhasana – Twist variation*

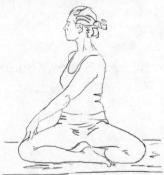

- Still sitting on your block or cushion, feel the crown of the head lift up directly over the sitting bones, inhale and twist to the right on the exhalation.

- Inhale space between each vertebra to avoid compression of spinal discs as you turn with the exhalation.
- Lift belly back and up to support your lower back, so the twist is felt between the shoulder blades and chest can lift.
- Keep the chin in line with the breastbone, collarbones broad.
- Inhale and turn to centre on the exhale.
- Settle, establish spinal length and repeat other side.

Marjaryasana/Bitilasana* – Cat/Cow Pose

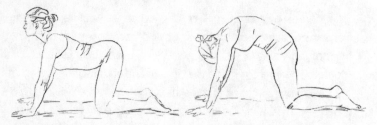

- From all fours, hands below the shoulders and knees under hips, with an exhalation, lift the spine up, dropping the head. With an inhalation, drop the spine between shoulders and hips.
- Let movement follow each breath right to its end-point.
- Continue for as many breaths as feels right and shoulders and spine fully loosen.

Adho Mukha Svanasana* – Down-face Dog

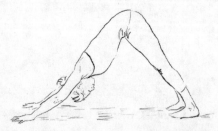

- From all fours, hands spread and middle fingers parallel, exhale as you lift bottom to the ceiling, heels up or legs slightly bent to start.

- Push back from the base of the index fingers to move the tops of the thighs back and lift the sitting bones.

- Suck in the side ribs and lengthen through the waist.

- Rather than forcing heels down, draw up the knees and allow the heels to move back and down as you push back from the palms.

- Stay as long as your breath is easy, then walk your feet towards your hands to Uttanasana. (If you're doing the shorter sequence, go straight to Balasana (page 214).

Uttanasana – Intense Stretch Pose

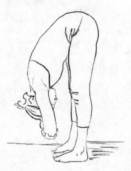

- Check your feet are hip-width apart, outer edges parallel. Hold elbows with opposite hands and hang from the hips.

- Strong legs create a soft lower back; draw up your kneecaps and drop into your heels to lift sitting bones to the sky.

- Gather muscles around the tops of the thigh bones and lift them up.

- Be mindful not to turn the feet out or lock the lower back. Bend your legs if you need to, without the knees 'knocking in'.

- Bend legs and roll up the spine to standing on an in-breath.

Tadasana – Mountain Pose

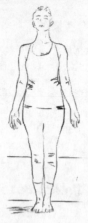

- Stand, feet together, balls of the feet and toes wide, and heels back to rise up from the floor to the crown of the head.
- Let your breath create trust in your body's ability to organize best posture, drawing the waist back and up to help.
- Drop down into broad heels, lifting insteps and gathering hips in together.
- Create awareness of all postural recommendations on pages 203–04.

Vrksasana – Tree Pose

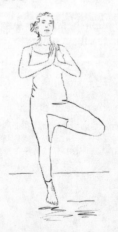

- While in Tadasana, find a steady focus point and then slowly move the weight onto the right foot, gathering in the right hip.
- Lift the left foot and place onto the inner thigh or inner calf. Bring your hands into prayer position at the heart.
- Press foot into leg and vice versa, and lift up from there to the crown of the head.
- Breathe into your focus point to balance.
- Bring the foot down to meet the other, settling in Tadasana before moving to the other side.

Uttanasana – as before, from standing hip-width apart

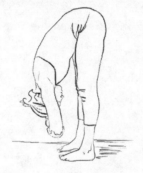

Adho Mukha Svanasana – as before, then sitting back onto the heels.

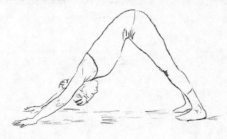

Vajrasana – Diamond Pose

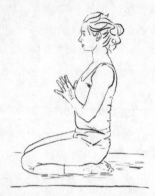

- Sitting with bottom on heels, drop down top thighs and lift the spine up. Put a block between the heels and buttocks if you need.
- Pull the waist back and up and lengthen the back of the neck.
- Bring the hands together into the heart for a point of breath focus.

Balasana* – Child Pose

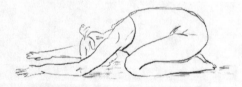

- From Vajrasana bring the big toes together, open the knees slightly apart and walk your hands forward to take your time to release the lower back and eventually bring the hairline to the floor or onto one or two blocks.
- Breathe into the tops of the thighs to release them down and anchor as the back of the pelvis broadens. Take as long as you need.
- Walk hands back towards knees, stacking up the spine to come up.

Supta Matsyendrasana – Supine Lord of the Fishes Pose*

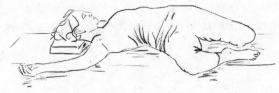

- Lie with head supported, legs bent. Walk your feet out to align the outer edges with edges of the mat.

- Open your arms out to a wide position, elbows comfortably bent. Inhale and then, on the exhalation, allow the knees to drop to the right side, rolling onto the sides of the feet.

- Let gravity take the weight of the legs down, release any gripping in the knees, breathing the spine long.

- Inhale back to centre (with pelvic floor support), then exhale down to the left. You can follow this flow several times before resting on each side in turn.

Setu Bandha Sarvangasana – Bridge Pose

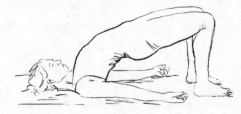

- Remove head support and lengthen neck, feet comfortably close to the buttocks, hip-width apart and little toe sides of the feet parallel, hands palm-up by the hips – settle the lower back here for at least 10 breaths.

- Inhale and lift the pelvis off the floor one vertebra at a time.

- Push back and up from the base of the big toe, roll the thighs in, flatten the belly and lift the breastbone strongly towards the chin.

- Stay as long as you can lift your chest with easy breath and soft face.
- Roll the spine down and rest until back muscles settle.

Supta Matsyendrasana – as before to release lower back

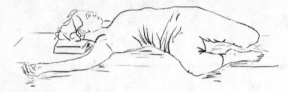

Savasana* – Corpse Pose

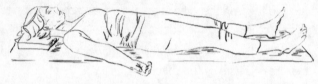

- Lie with your head on a block or cushion to quiet your mind. With arms comfortably away from the body, lift each shoulder blade down the body to open the chest.
- Stay for 2–3 minutes minimum – 10 minutes is optimal when you have enough time, practising breathing to cultivate awareness and full relaxation.
- Bend your legs and roll onto your side, lie for a few breaths before making a smooth transition into your day.

Evening Practice

Our bodies can be more open in the evening than in the morning after daily movement, so flexibility comes more easily, helping you wind down and release the day. You'll see many poses here described as 'restorative'. This is a specific practice where the body is positioned so it has to exert no muscular force. You need to be able to relax fully in these postures, so if there is any pain or discomfort, move or support as described to relieve it, but also give yourself a chance to settle in with the breath and see how your body responds as it lets go of stress.

You may feel deep and unfamiliar sensations as you release. Practising non-reaction with a calm mind helps us to discern between safe but intense feelings of postural change and sharp, shooting or non-subsiding pain, which is a signal to be listened to. Find the bodily comfort that allows you to come to that alpha, meditative state. You can stay in restorative poses for up to 20 minutes and the focus should be on any aspect of breath we have described. Our nervous systems take at least 15 minutes of full relaxation to reach a true *somatic* state where we can fully recuperate.

If you want a longer practice and feel the need to move through some tension or nervous energy from the day, you can start with the morning practice, coming down with the full evening sequence afterwards, or even spend just 15 minutes or so in one or two of the following restorative postures. You know your energy, routine and stresses will be different on different days, so use your intuition to help find and choose the best options for you. Variety and adaptability are two more great reasons yoga works in everyday life.

If you need something simple or short that you can fully surrender in to, we have highlighted *Evening Priority poses**,* as one or two of these can ensure that you fully engage the relaxing parasympathetic nervous system to take you towards sleep. Charlotte often simply does a long Pavanamuktasana, Jathara Parivartanasana and then Savasana for evening practice.

Pavanamuktasana** – Wind-relieving Pose, restorative

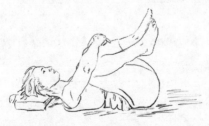

- Start from lying with soles of the feet on the floor, legs bent, skull supported by a block or cushion.

- Draw the knees up into the chest, looping the arms around shins or backs of thighs, holding the fingers of one hand with the other.
- Allow the knees to drop open towards the armpits and the weight of the legs to start opening the hips over time.
- Drop the feet to the floor, roll to one side and lie comfortably in the foetal position before coming up.

Siddhasana – Adept's Pose – forward bend, restorative variation to chair

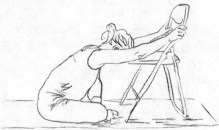

- Facing a chair in Siddhasana (see Morning Practice), breathe until the hips settle.
- Lengthen the spine by reaching to the back or sides of the chair, eventually resting the forehead on the chair seat (with optional cushion) with arms extended or folded on the seat – move the chair if you need: forward as you release more over time.
- Drop into the sitting bones to safely release back muscles.
- Press into the chair to sit up for a few moments before changing the cross of the legs and repeating.

Adho Mukha Svanasana – as Morning Practice

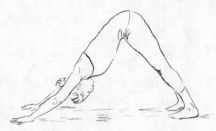

Vajrasana – as Morning Practice

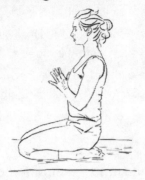

Balasana – as Morning Practice, restorative version

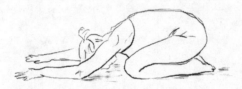

- To stay longer in child pose, you can support the head and torso with a bolster or couple of pillows, turning the head to face each side for an equal amount of time.

*Jathara Parivartanasana** – Revolved Abdomen Pose, restorative version*

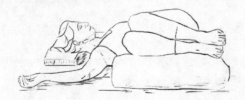

- Have a bolster or stack of towels ready to support your legs by your right ribs, skull supported with block or cushion.

- Open your arms out to a wide position with elbows comfortably bent, backs of hands easily touching the floor, front shoulders soft.
- With knees into the chest, inhale to lift pelvis and exhale to drop the legs to the right fully onto the support.
- As you release, broaden collarbones and revolve ribcage away from the legs to allow the left shoulder to drop as the chest opens.
- Inhale legs to centre, exhale to floor, rest and repeat other side.

Supta Baddha Konasana** – Supine Bound Angle Pose, restorative

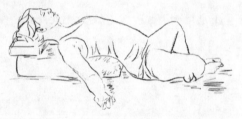

- Move your bolster/towels (your 'lift') lengthways on your mat, cushion or block at the far end for your head.
- Sit with soles of the feet together, close into groin, about a fist-width in front of your lift. Press hands down either side of your hips to lift your pelvis, contract belly to strongly tuck under tail-bone, holding as you drop your bottom back down. Lie over your lift, with neck comfortable, arms as in Savasana.
- If there is any pinching in the lower back, move the buttocks down to create length. Support thighs equally with cushions if necessary. Breathe easily, with eyes closed, focus internal.
- To come out, tuck chin firmly into chest, press down into floor with hands and come up on one in-breath.

*Viparita Karani** – Waterfall Practice, restorative*

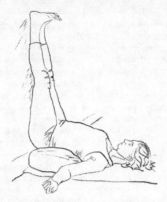

- Position your lift parallel and a couple of inches away from a wall.
- Sit on the end of your lift, lower hip close to the wall and swing legs up. Shimmy your lower back fully onto the lift, whole of your pelvis supported but not digging into the waist. Lie with arms as in Savasana, or over your head if comfortable for the shoulders.
- If you have tight hamstrings, move lift further away from the wall.
- Roll off your lift with one breath, lying in a foetal position to relax before coming up.

*Savasana** – as Morning Practice, always restorative*

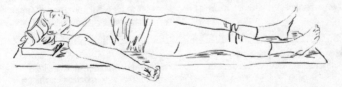

- Option to support the legs with a bolster or rolled blanket under the knees. Place an eye pillow or scarf over your eyes to cut out the light and cover yourself with a blanket to feel the full De-Stress effects of being cocooned and safe.

Yoga Practice by Stress Suit

	You may find that you...	Best Single Change You Could Make
Stressed and Wired	feel frustrated by not being able to get into that stronger/harder/ bendier position	'Flexibility envy' is a term bandied about by yoga teachers, as an aid to help keep ambition and ego in check. More force means more tension and less likelihood of a deep stretch, so focus on breathing.
Stressed and Tired	tend to want to just lie down and drift off	Yes, restorative positions do just that, but also use more energizing poses to encourage good oxygenation to help reduce fatigue, and twists to support the adrenal glands.
Stressed and Cold	feel pain, tingling, numbness or pins and needles when you practise	Opening the throat and increasing circulation around the upper chest and thyroid is beneficial for you. Breathe into these sensations coming up as circulation improves.
Stressed and Bloated	find it difficult to connect to belly breathing and postural support as your abdomen tends to swell	Twists, with an emphasis on creating length in the waist, give the intestines and bowel a good massage and improve detoxification. Breathe lying down to allow the diaphragm to move and abdominal contents to relax.
Stressed and Sore	feel pain or tightness in joints when you move into postures	Check that all postures are safe for you with a doctor or osteopath. Pain that changes when you move tends to be structural but continual whatever your position is often more inflammatory.
Stressed and Demotivated	intend to but ultimately can't be bothered to start a yoga practice	Start small: even 5 minutes of Cat/Cow, Down-face Dog, Balasana, one of the floor twists and then Savasana will have positive effects and motivate you to continue.
Stressed and Hormonal	feel vast differences in your postures at different times of the month	Supta Baddha Konasana is the ultimate PMS and hormonal pose, bringing circulation and connection to the groin area. Differences are the best guide for connecting with what you need at any given time.

Chapter 12
PROGRESS TOOLS

The charts in this section are designed to help you keep a record of your progress as you embark upon your journey to a healthier, slimmer, calmer you. They are available to download and print out within the De-Stress 6-Week Support Plan at de-stressyourlife.com

1. **Daily Living Chart** – a complete picture of a De-Stress day to help you change old habits.

2. **What to Eat** – an overview of the De-Stress Diet to help guide change.

3. **Changing Your Food Habits** – for noting down what might need changing and at a level you decide.

4. **Energy, Mood and Appetite** – helping you to work out which foods and lifestyle choices make you feel best, and will suit your De-Stress health and weight-loss goals long term.

Use these for:
*   learning and memory tools as you start out on your De-Stress journey
*   help in deciding your levels of progressive change and noting how they made you feel
*   guides to help you get back should you have an off-day
*   reflective diaries for charting what suits you long term
*   occasional 'check-ins' to take the 'stress temperature' of your life.

De-Stress Progress Chart – Daily Living

Page ref.	Which De-Stress action are you including this week?	Personal notes
	Starting your day:	
86	Lemon in hot water	
87	Breakfast with protein	
66–68, 95	Morning supplements	
195–98	Mindful eating/breathing awareness	
11	Cold at end of shower	
169–76, 207–16	Yoga/walk/exercise	
169–77	De-Stress strength-training routine	
	Daytime working day:	
117–21	Eat lunch away from desk/ workplace	
195–98	Mindful eating/breathing awareness	
177–78	Spontaneous activity/walking	
113, 186–87	Sunlight exposure	
195	10 deep breaths during stress	
	Daytime day off:	
112	A long, luxurious lunch	
195–98	Mindful eating/breathing awareness	
177–78	Spontaneous activity/walking	
169–77	De-Stress strength-training routine	
113, 186–87	Sunlight exposure	
195	10 deep breaths during stress	
184–86	Socializing/group activity	
	Evening:	
126	Early evening exercise	
169–77	De-Stress strength-training routine	
132	Dinner at a reasonable time	
195–98	Mindful eating/breathing awareness	
127, 136–38	Any sleep supplements/natural aids	
195–200, 216–21	Yoga/breathing/meditation	
184–86	Laughter with friends/socializing	
124	Little electronic stimulus	
125	Reasonable sleep time	

Mon	Tue	Wed	Thu	Fri	Sat	Sun

De-Stress Progress Chart – What to Eat

Page ref.	Highlight which De-Stress dietary inclusion you are focusing on this week:	Personal notes
	Mealtimes:	
46–48, 58	Protein with every meal	
50–52, 58–59	Healthy fats	
60	Bitter foods	
60	Thermogenic foods	
	Vegetables included:	
	Raw and cooked	
	Dark green leafy veg	
59	Cruciferous veg	
	Allowed root veg	
	Garlic and onions	
	Fruit:	
	2 portions a day	
	3 to help initial sugar weaning	
149	None to help wean off sweet tastes	
	Cause bloating after protein meal	
	Snacking habits:	
140	None	
141–43	Need between breakfast and lunch	
141–43	Need between lunch and dinner	
147–48	Late night pudding or cravings	
	Non-caffeine or alcohol fluid intake:	
150	More fluids between meals	
152–56	Caffeine only after food	
151	Rehydrating apple juice/water or coconut water	

Mon	Tue	Wed	Thu	Fri	Sat	Sun

De-Stress Progress Chart – Changing Your Food Habits

Page ref.	Highlight which De-Stress action you are including this week:	Personal notes
140 141–43 63–64, 73–5 147–48	**Snacking habits:** None Need between breakfast and lunch Need between lunch and dinner Late night pudding or cravings	
32 52–53 64–66	**Dairy:** Complete avoidance this phase Occasional	
49–50 63–64 76–78 32	**Grains:** Complete avoidance this phase Just sourdough rye breakfast or lunch Occasional with lunch only Avoiding gluten grains	
49–50 63–64 76–77 110–11	**Beans:** Complete avoidance this phase Occasional with lunch or dinner Including beans as vegetarian or vegan – cooking as advised	
48 76–77 63–64	**Potatoes, sweet potatoes, parsnips, yams:** Complete avoidance Small portion late night stops bingeing	
73–75 148–49 147–48 78–79	**Sugar avoidance:** Avoiding completely Daily 40mg dark chocolate for weaning Able to cope with occasional treats	
152–56	**Caffeine:** None 2 cups maximum coffee or tea Switching to green tea Weaning off as agitates	
156–59 78–79	**Alcohol:** None Occasional treat	

Mon	Tue	Wed	Thu	Fri	Sat	Sun

De-Stress Progress Chart – Energy, Mood and Appetite

Note the changes you have made, and when, in the column below, then how you felt afterwards at relevant times in columns to the right. Do this for several days to see how evening affects sleep and the next morning, and the effects over 3- to 4-day cycles:	On waking	Mid-morning	Lunchtime
Note any new foods eaten: 1. 2. 3. 4.			
Note any grains, beans, dairy, potatoes, sweet potatoes, parsnips or yams eaten: 1. 2. 3.			
Note any sugar sources eaten or drunk and/or reductions: 1. 2. 3.			
Note any weaning off caffeine progress: 1. 2. 3.			
Note any healthy food or drinks used to help energy and relief from cravings: 1. 2. 3.			
Note any changes in alcohol intake: 1. 2. 3.			
Note any increase in non-caffeinated or non-alcoholic fluids: 1. 2. 3.			

Mid-afternoon	Early evening	Late evening	Sleep quality

REFERENCES

Introduction

1. European Agency for Safety and Health at Work, 'Stress at Work – Facts and Figures', European Risk Observatory Report, 2009
2. Reay, G, Iddon, B. *Report by All Party Parliamentary Drugs Misuse Group: Inquiry into Physical Dependence and Addiction to Prescription and Over-the-Counter Drugs 2008–2009*
3. *Skillsoft Report: Research into UK Workers Stress Levels* online survey 2008; accessed August 2011
4. Professor Carol Shively in interview with Anna Magee, quoted with kind permission
5. Shively, C A, Wallace, J. 'Social Status, Social Stress and Fat Distribution in Primates', *International Textbook of Obesity* (John Wiley & Sons, 2001)
6. Tapper, K. *et al.* 'Exploratory randomised controlled trial of a mindfulness-based weight loss intervention for women', *Appetite* 2009; 52(2): 396–404
7. Smith, B W. 'A Preliminary Study of the Effects of a Modified Mindfulness Intervention on Binge Eating', *Journal of Evidence-Based Complementary & Alternative Medicine* 2006; 11(3): 133–43
8. Kristeller, J L. 'An Exploratory Study of a Meditation-based Intervention for Binge Eating Disorder', *J Health Psychol.* 1999; 4(3): 357–63
9. Baer, R A. *Mindfulness-Based Treatment Approaches: A clinician's guide to evidence base and applications* (Academic Press, 2005)

Chapter 1 – Why Stress Makes You Fat and Unhealthy

1. Mann, T *et al.* 'Medicare's Search for Effective Obesity Treatments', *American Psychologist* 2007: 221–33
2. World Health Organization, *Obesity and Overweight Factsheet*, March 2011
3. Sapolsky, R M. *Why Zebras Don't Get Ulcers* (Holt, 2004)
4. Mattson, M P. 'Hormesis Defined', *Ageing Res. Rev.* 2008; 7(1): 1–7
5. Dr Mark Mattson in interview with Anna Magee, quoted with kind permission
6. Huether, G *et al.* 'The stress-reaction process and the adaptive modification and reorganization of neuronal networks', *Psychiatry Research* 1999; 87(1): 83–95
7. Professor Leo Puimboom, Globesity Seminar 2011, quoted with kind permission
8. Block, J P *et al.* 'Psychosocial Stress and Change in Weight Among US Adults', *Am. J. Epidemiol.* 2009; 170(2): 181–92

9. Chandola, T et al. 'Chronic stress at work and the metabolic syndrome: prospective study' BMJ 2006; 332: 521

10. Shively, C A, Wallace, J. 'Social Status, Social Stress and Fat Distribution in Primates', International Textbook of Obesity (John Wiley & Sons, 2001)

11. Kudielko, B M et al. 'HPA Axis responses to laboratory psychosocial stress in healthy elderly adults, younger adults and children', Psychoneuroimmunology 2004; 29(1): 83–98

12. Epel, E S et al. 'Stress may add bite to appetite in women: a laboratory study of stress-induced cortisol and eating behavior', Psychoneuroendocrinology 2001; 26(1): 37–49

13. Epel, E S et al. 'Stress and body shape: stress-induced cortisol secretion is consistently greater among women with central fat', Psychosomatic Medicine 2000; 62: 623–32

14. Park, A. 'Fat Bellied Monkeys Suggest Why Stress Sucks', Time Magazine August 8, 2009.

15. Debigare, R et al. 'Catabolic/Anabolic Balance and Muscle Wasting in Patients with COPD', Chest 2003; 124(1): 83–89

16. Falconer, I R et al. 'Effect of adrenal hormones on thyroid secretion and thyroid hormones on adrenal secretion in the sheep', J Physiol. 1975; 250(2): 261–73

17. Pecina, S et al. 'Nucleus accumbenscorticotropin-releasing factor increases cue-triggered motivation for sucrose reward: paradoxical positive incentive effects in stress?', BMC Biology 2006; 4: 8

18. Epel, E S et al. 'Stress may add bite to appetite in women: a laboratory study of stress-induced cortisol and eating behavior', Psychoneuroendocrinology 2001; 26(1): 37–49

19. George, S A et al. 'CRH-stimulated cortisol release and food intake in healthy, non-obese adults', Psychoneuroendocrinology 2010; 35(4): 607–12

20. Neim, N L et al. 'Relation between circulating leptin concentrations and appetite during a prolonged, moderate energy deficit in women', American Journal of Clinical Nutrition 1998; 68: 794–801

21. Wang, G et al. 'Gastric stimulation in obese subjects activates the hippocampus and other regions involved in brain reward circuitry', Proceedings of the National Academy of Science 2006; 103(42): 15641–45

22. Adam, T C et al. 'Stress, eating and the reward system', Physiology & Behaviour 2007; 91(4): 449–458

23. Krebs, H et al. 'Effects of stressful noise on eating and non-eating behavior in rats', Appetite 1996; 26(2): 193–202

24. Strack, F et al. 'Reflective and Impulsive Determinants of Social Behaviour', Personality and Social Psychology Review 2004; 8(3): 220–47

25. Baumeister, R F et al. 'The Strength Model of Self Control', Current Directions in Psychological Science 2007; 16(6): 351–55

26. Hofmann, W, Friese, M. 'Control Yourself!' Scientific American Mind, May/June 2011: 43–47

Chapter 2 – Which Stress Suit Are You Wearing?

1. McEwan, B. 'Protective and damaging effects of stress mediators', NEJM 1998; 338(3): 171–79

2. Kyrou, I et al. 'Stress, visceral obesity, and metabolic complications', Ann NY Acad Sci 2006; 1083: 77110

3. *What is Functional Medicine?* The Institute for Functional Medicine http://www.functionalmedicine.org/about/whatis.asp accessed August 2011

4. Weatherby, D. *Signs and Symptoms Analysis from a Functional Perspective* (2nd edn; Weatherby & Associates, LLC 2004)

5. Pizzorno, J E, Murray, M T. *Textbook of Natural Medicine* (3rd edn; Churchill Livingstone, 2010)

6. Pruessner, J C et al. 'Burnout, perceived stress, and cortisol responses to awakening', *Psychosom Med* 1999; 61(2): 197–204

7. Anderson, D C. 'Assessment and nutraceutical management of stress-induced adrenal dysfunction', *Integrative Medicine* 2008; 7(5): 18–25

8. Mohler, H. 'GABA$_A$ Receptors in Central Nervous System Disease: Anxiety, Epilepsy, and Insomnia', *Journal of Receptors and Signal Transduction* 2006; 26(5–6): 731–40

9. Wilson, J. *Adrenal Fatigue, the 21st Century Stress Syndrome* (Smart Publications, 2002)

10. Ko, F N et al. 'Vasodilatory action mechanisms of apigenin isolated from Apium-graveolens in rat thoracic aorta', *BiochimBiophysActa* 1991; 1115(1): 69–74

11. Ruston, D et al. 'The National Diet and Nutrition Survey: adults aged 19 to 64 years' (Volume 4; HMSO, 2004)

12. Pohl, H R et al. 'Metal ions affecting the neurological system', *Met Ions Life Sci* 2011; 8: 247–62

13. Toyama, T. 'Isothiocyanates Reduce Mercury Accumulation via an Nrf2-Dependent Mechanism during Exposure of Mice to Methylmercury', *Environ Health Perspect* 2011; 119(8): 1117–22

14. Fries, E et al. 'A new view on hypocortisolism', *Psychoneuroendocrinology* 2005; 30(10): 1010–16

15. Miller, G E et al. 'If it goes up, must it come down? Chronic stress and the hypothalamic–pituitary–adrenocortical axis in humans', *Psychol Bull* 2007; 133(1): 25–45

16. Heim, C et al. 'The potential role of hypocortisolism in the pathophysiology of stress-related bodily disorders', *Psychoneuroendocrinology* 2000; 25(1): 1–35

17. Oelkers, W. 'Adrenal insufficiency', *NEJM*; 335 (16): 1206–12

18. Scherrer, U, Sartori, C. 'Insulin as a vascular and sympathoexcitatory hormone', *Circulation* 1997; 96: 4104–13

19. 'Progression of Stages of Adrenal Exhaustion' (BioHealth Diagnostics, 2004)

20. Swain, M G, et al. 'Fatigue in Chronic disease', *Clinical Science* 2000; 99: 1–8

21. Neustadt, J. 'Mitochondrial dysfunction and disease', *Integrative Medicine* 2006; 5(3): 14–20

22. Office of Dietary Supplements. *Dietary Supplement Fact Sheet: Iron* (Health Professional). US National Institutes of Health http://ods.od.nih.gov/factsheets/Iron–HealthProfessional accessed August 2011

23. Ortancil, O et al. 'Association between serum ferritin level and fibromyalgia syndrome', *Eur J ClinNutr* 2010; 64(3): 308–12

24. Brzozowska, M et al. 'Evaluation of influence of selenium, copper, zinc and iron concentrations on thyroid gland size in school children with normal ioduria', *Pol MerkurLekarski* 2006; 20(120): 672–77

25. Pullakhandam, R et al. 'Bioavailability of iron and zinc from multiple micronutrient fortified beverage premixes in Caco-2 cell model', *J Food Sci* 2011; 76(2): H38–42

26. Kim, E Y et al. 'Ascorbic acid offsets the inhibitory effect of bioactive dietary

polyphenolic compounds on transepithelial iron transport in Caco–2 intestinal cells', *J Nutr* 2011; 141(5): 828–34

27. Office of Dietary Supplements. *Dietary Supplement Fact Sheet: Vitamin B12* (Health Professional). US National Institutes of Health http://ods.od.nih.gov/factsheets/VitaminB12–HealthProfessional accessed August 2011

28. Norris, J, Messina, G. 'B12 in Tempeh, Seaweeds, Organic Produce, and Other Plant Foods', http://www.veganhealth.org/b12/plant accessed August 2011

29. Allen, L H. 'Bioavailability of vitamin B$_{12}$', *Int J VitamNutr Res* 2010; 80(4–5): 330–35

30. Charmandari, E et al. 'Pediatric stress: hormonal mediators and human development', *Horm Res* 2003; 59(4): 161–79

31. SaitGonen, M et al. 'Assessment of anxiety in subclinical thyroid disorders', *Endocrine Journal* 2004; 51(3): 311–15

32. Durrant-Peatfield, B. 'Adrenal and Thyroid Gland Testing and Protocols', lecture notes attended Genova Diagnostics 2005

33. Son, H Y et al. 'Synergistic interaction between excess caffeine and deficient iodine on the promotion of thyroid carcinogenesis in rats pretreated with N–bis(2–hydroxypropyl)nitrosamine', *Cancer Sci* 2003; 94(4): 334–37

34. Vanderpas, J. 'Nutritional epidemiology and thyroid hormone metabolism', *Annu. Rev. Nutr* 2006; 26: 293–322

35. Verhoeven, D T et al. 'A review of mechanisms underlying anticarcinogenicity by brassica vegetables', *Chem. Biol. Interact* 1997; 103(2): 79–129

36. Triggiani, V et al. 'Role of iodine, selenium and other micronutrients in thyroid function and disorders', *EndocrMetab Immune Disord Drug Targets* 2009; 9(3): 277

37. Brzozowska, M et al. 'Evaluation of influence of selenium, copper, zinc and iron concentrations on thyroid gland size in school children with normal ioduria', *Pol MerkurLekarski* 2006; 20(120): 672–77

38. Medline Plus. 'Iodine in diet', US National Institutes of Health http://www.nlm.nih.gov/medlineplus/ency/article/002421.htm accessed August 2011

39. Lee, S. 'Iodine Deficiency', Medscape Reference http://emedicine.medscape.com/article/122714–overview accessed August 2011

40. Office of Dietary Supplements. *Dietary Supplement Fact Sheet: Iodine* (Health Professional). US National Institutes of Health http://ods.od.nih.gov/factsheets/Iodine–HealthProfessional accessed August 2011

41. International Council for Control of Iodine Deficiency Disorders. *IDD Newsletter* 2008; 29(3)

42. Zimmermann, M B. 'Iodine deficiency', *Endocr Rev* 2009; 30(4): 376–408

43. Speeckaert, M M et al. 'Value and pitfalls in iodine fortification and supplementation in the 21st century', *Br J Nutr* 2011; 4: 1–10

44. Collins, S M, Bercik, P. 'The relationship between intestinal microbiota and the central nervous system in normal gastrointestinal function and disease', *Gastroenterology* 2009; 136(6): 2003–14

45. Lyte, M. et al. 'Induction of anxiety-like behavior in mice during the initial stages of infection with the agent of murine colonic hyperplasia Citrobacterrodentium', *PhysiolBehav* 2006; 89(3): 350–57

46. Knowles, S R et al. 'Investigating the role of perceived stress on bacterial flora activity and salivary cortisol secretion: a possible mechanism underlying susceptibility to illness', *BiolPsychol* 2008; 77(2): 132–37

47. Hawrelak, J A, Myers, S P. 'The causes of intestinal dysbiosis: a review', *Altern Med Rev* 2004; 9(2): 180–97

48. Lutgendorff, F *et al*. 'The role of microbiota and probiotics in stress-induced gastro-intestinal damage', *CurrMol Med* 2008; 8(4): 282–98

49. Ash, M. *A Novel Approach to Treating Depression – How Probiotics Can Shift Mood by Modulating Cytokines* (Nutri-Link Ltd–Clinical Education, 2009)

50. Kirkham, M, Martin, S. 'Eat less, chew more: getting the basics right for successful treatment', *CAM* 2005: 26–31

51. Hughes, C. 'Galactooligosaccharide supplementation reduces stress-induced gastrointestinal dysfunction and days of cold or flu: a randomized, double-blind, controlled trial in healthy university students', *Am J ClinNutr* 2011; 93(6): 1305–11

52. Parnell, J A. 'Weight loss during oligofructose supplementation is associated with decreased ghrelin and increased peptide YY in overweight and obese adults', *Am J ClinNutr* 2009; 89(6): 1751–59

53. Francis, C Y. 'Bran and irritable bowel syndrome: time for reappraisal' *The Lancet* 1994; 344(8914): 39–40

54. Drago, S. 'Gliadin, zonulin and gut permeability: Effects on celiac and non-celiac intestinal mucosa and intestinal cell lines', *Scandinavian Journal of Gastroenterology* 2006; 41(4): 408–19

55. Dolfini, E. 'Damaging effects of gliadin on three-dimensional cell culture model', *World J Gastroenterol* 2005; 11(3): 5973–77

56. Auricchio, S *et al*. 'Gluten-sensitive enteropathy in childhood', *PediatrClin North Am* 1988; 35(1): 157–87

57. Jönsson, T *et al*. 'Agrarian diet and diseases of affluence – Do evolutionary novel dietary lectins cause leptin resistance?', *BMC Endocrine Disorders* 2005; 5: 10

58. Dixit, V, Mak, T W. 'NF–kappa B signalling. Many roads lead to Madrid', *Cell* 2002; 111: 615–19

59. Lee, D F, Hung, M C. 'All roads lead to m-TOR: integrating inflammation and tumor angiogenesis', *Cell Cycle* 2007; 6: 3011–14

60. Harbuz, M *et al*. 'Hypothalamo–pituitary–adrenal axis and chronic immune activation', *Ann NY Acad Sci* 2003; 992, 99–106

61. Padgett, D A, Glaser, R. 'How stress influences the immune response' *Trends Immunol* 2003; 24(8): 444–48

62. Epel, E S *et al*. 'Accelerated telomere shortening in response to life stress', *ProcNatlAcadSci USA* 2004; 101(49): 17312–15

63. Harbuz, M *et al*. 'Hypothalamo–pituitary–adrenal axis and chronic immune activation', *Ann NY Acad Sci* 2003; 992: 99–106

64. Khaustova, S A *et al*. 'Short highly intense exercise causes changes in salivary concentrations of hydrocortisone and secretory IgA', *Bull Exp Biol* 2010; 149(5): 635–39

65. Elenkov, I J, Chrousos, G P. 'Stress, cytokine patterns and susceptibility to disease', *ClinEndocrinolMetab* 1999; 13(4): 583–95

66. Sivamani, R *et al*. 'Stress-mediated increases in systemic and local epinephrine impair skin wound healing: Potential new indication for beta blockers', *PLoS* 2009; 6(1): e12

67. Raison, C L *et al*. 'Interferon–alpha effects on diurnal hypothalamic–pituitary–adrenal axis activity: relationship with proinflammatory cytokines and behavior', *Mol Psychiatry* 2010; 15(5): 535–47

References

68. Robels, T F et al. 'Out of Balance: A New Look at Chronic Stress, Depression, and Immunity', Current Directions in Psychological Science 2005; 14(2): 111–15

69. Meier, U, Gressner, A M. 'Endocrine Regulation of Energy Metabolism: Review of Pathobiochemical and Clinical Chemical Aspects of Leptin, Ghrelin, Adiponectin, and Resistin', Clinical Chemistry 2004; 50(9): 1511–25

70. Elliott, W. 'Criterion validity of a computer-based tutorial for teaching waist circumference self-measurement', Journal of Bodywork and Movement Therapies 2008; 12(2): 133–45

71. Sharma, A M. 'Adipose tissue: a mediator of cardiovascular risk', Int J ObesRelat Meta Disord 2002; 26(4): S5–7

72. Melpomeni, P et al. 'Glucose, Advanced Glycation End Products, and Diabetes Complications: What Is New and What Works', Clinical Diabetes 2003; 21(4): 186–87

73. Simopoulos, A P. 'The Mediterranean Diets: What Is So Special about the Diet of Greece? The Scientific Evidence', J. Nutr 2001; 131: 3065S–3073S

74. Freed, D L F. 'Do dietary lectins cause disease? The evidence is suggestive – and raises interesting possibilities for treatment', BMJ 1999; 318(7190): 1023–1024

75. Gupta, Y P. 'Antinutritional and toxic factors in food legumes: a review', Plant Foods for Human Nutrition 1987; 37: 201–28

76. Cordain, L et al. 'Modulation of immune function by dietary lectins in rheumatoid arthritis', Br J Nutr 2000; 83(3): 207–17

77. James, M et al. 'Fish oil and rheumatoid arthritis: past, present and future', ProcNutr Soc 2010; 69: 316–23

78. Wall, R et al. 'Fatty acids from fish: the anti-inflammatory potential of long-chain fatty acids', Nutr Rev 2010; 68: 280–89

79. Leonard, B E. 'The HPA and immune axes in stress: the involvement of the serotonergic system', Eur Psychiatry 2005; 20: S302–306

80. Rada, P et al. 'Daily bingeing on sugar repeatedly releases dopamine in the accumbens shell', Neuroscience 2005; 134(3): 737–44

81. Dallman, M F. 'Stress-induced obesity and the emotional nervous system', Trends EndocrinolMetab 2010; 21(3): 159–65

82. Avena, N M. 'Examining the addictive-like properties of binge eating using an animal model of sugar dependence', ExpClinPsychopharmacol 2007; 15(5): 481–91

83. Warne, J P. 'Shaping the stress response: interplay of palatable food choices, glucocorticoids, insulin and abdominal obesity', Mol Cell Endocrinol 2009; 300(1–2): 137–46

84. Shelton, R C, Miller, A H. 'Eating ourselves to death (and despair): the contribution of adiposity and inflammation to depression' ProgNeurobiol 2010; 91(4): 275–99

85. Pecoraro, N et al. 'Chronic stress promotes palatable feeding, which reduces signs of stress: feedforward and feedback effects of chronic stress', Endocrinology 2004; 145(8): 3754–62

86. Raison, C L et al. 'Cytokines sing the blues: inflammation and the pathogenesis of depression', TrendsImmunol 2006; 27(1): 24–31

87. Swenne, I. 'Omega–3 polyunsaturated essential fatty acids are associated with depression in adolescents with eating disorders and weight loss', ActaPaediatr 2011 [Epub ahead of print]

88. Office of Dietary Supplements. Dietary Supplement Fact Sheet: Vitamin D (Health Professional). US National Institutes of Health http://ods.od.nih.gov/factsheets/vitamind#h5 accessed August 2011

89. Vanoirbeek, E et al. 'The anti-cancer and anti-inflammatory actions of 1,25(OH)(2) D(3)', Best Pract Res ClinEndocrinolMetab 2011; 25(4): 593–604

90. Lips, P, van Schoor, N M. 'The effect of vitamin D on bone and osteoporosis', Best Pract Res ClinEndocrinolMetab 2011; 25(4): 585–91

91. Cherniack, E P et al. 'Some new food for thought: the role of vitamin D in the mental health of older adults', Curr Psychiatry Rep 2009; 11(1): 12–19

92. Van Schoor, N M, Lips, P. 'Worldwide vitamin D status', Best Pract Res ClinEndocrinolMetab 2011; 25(4): 671–80

93. Walf, A A, Frye, C A. 'Review and Update of Mechanisms of Estrogen in the Hippocampus and Amygdala for Anxiety and Depression Behavior', Neuropsychopharmacology 2006; 31: 1097–1111

94. Textbook of Functional Medicine (Institute for Functional Medicine, 2005): 229

95. Glenville, M. Mastering Cortisol: Stop Your Body's Stress Hormone from Making You Fat Around the Middle (Amorata Press, 2006)

96. Touillaud, M S et al. 'Dietary lignan intake and postmenopausal breast cancer risk by oestrogen and progesterone receptor status', J Natl Cancer Inst 2007; 99(6): 475–867

97. Shu, X O et al. 'Soy food intake and breast cancer survival', JAMA 2009; 302(22): 2437–43

98. Liener, I E. 'Implications of antinutritional components in soybean foods', Crit Rev Food SciNutr 1994; 34: 31–67

99. Gold, E B et al. 'Diet and lifestyle associated with premenstrual symptoms in a racially diverse community sample: Study of Women's Health Across the Nation (SWAN)', J Womens Health 2007; 16(5): 641–56

100. Kavlock, R J et al. 'Research needs for the risk assessment of health and environmental effects of endocrine disruptors: A report of the U.S. EPA-sponsored workshop', Environ. Health Perspect 1996; 104(4): 715–40

101. Malekinejad, H et al. 'Naturally occurring oestrogens in processed milk and in raw milk (from gestated cows)', J Agric Food Chem 2006; 54(26): 9785–91

Chapter 3 – Slim and Calm on a Plate: De-Stress Diet Overview

1. Carrera-Bastos, P et al. 'The western diet and lifestyle and diseases of civilization', Res Rep ClinCardiol 2011; 2: 215–35

2. Chahwan, R. 'The Multidimensional Nature of Epigenetic Information and Its Role in Disease', Discov Med 2011; 58: 233–43

3. Frassetto, L A et al. 'Metabolic and physiologic improvements from consuming a paleolithic, hunter-gatherer type diet', Eur J ClinNutr 2009; 63(8): 947–55

4. O'Keefe, J H et al. 'Achieving hunter-gatherer fitness in the 21st century: back to the future', Am J Med 2010; 123(12): 1082–86

5. Johnson, J B et al. 'The effect on health of alternate day calorie restriction: eating less and more than needed on alternate days prolongs life', Med Hypothese 2006; 67(2): 209–11

6. Simopoulos, A P. 'The Mediterranean Diets: What Is So Special about the Diet of Greece? The Scientific Evidence', J. Nutr 2001; 131: 3065S–3073S

7. Cordain, L. 'The nutritional characteristics of a contemporary diet based upon Paleolithic food groups', J Am Nutraceut Assoc 2002; 5: 15–24

8. Henderson, L et al. 'The National Diet and Nutrition Survey: adults aged 19 to 64 years' (Volume 3; HMSO, 2003)

9. Jönsson, T et al. 'Beneficial effects of a Paleolithic diet on cardiovascular risk factors in type 2 diabetes: a randomized cross-over pilot study', CardiovascDiabetol 2009; 8: 35

10. Simopoulos, A P. 'The Mediterranean Diets: What Is So Special about the Diet of Greece? The Scientific Evidence', J. Nutr 2001; 131: 3065S–3073S

11. O'Dea, K. 'Marked improvement in carbohydrate and lipid metabolism in diabetic Australian aborigines after temporary reversion to traditional lifestyle', Diabetes 1984; 33(6): 596–603

12. Osterdahl, M et al. 'Effects of a short-term intervention with a paleolithic diet in healthy volunteers', Eur J ClinNutr 2008; 62(5): 682–85

13. Cordain, L et al. 'Origins and evolution of the Western diet: health implications for the 21st century', Am J ClinNutr 2005; 81(2): 341–54

14. Jönsson, T et al. 'A Paleolithic diet confers higher insulin sensitivity, lower C-reactive protein and lower blood pressure than a cereal-based diet in domestic pigs', NutrMetab (Lond) 2006; 3: 39

15. Carrera-Bastos, P et al. 'The western diet and lifestyle and diseases of civilization', Res Rep ClinCardiol 2011; 2: 215–35

16. Henderson, L et al. 'The National Diet and Nutrition Survey: adults aged 19 to 64 years' (Volume 2; HMSO, 2003)

17. Henderson, L et al. 'The National Diet and Nutrition Survey: adults aged 19 to 64 years' (Volume 1; HMSO, 2002)

18. Frank, B H. 'Are refined carbohydrates worse than saturated fat?', Am J ClinNutr 2010; 91(6): 1541–42

19. Hite, A H et al. 'In the face of contradictory evidence: Report of the Dietary Guidelines for Americans Committee', Nutrition 2010; 26(10): 915–24

20. Yin, X et al. 'Ghrelin fluctuation, what determines its production?', ActaBiochimBiophys Sin 2009; 41(3): 188–97

21. Feinma, R D. '"A calorie is a calorie" violates the second law of thermodynamics', Nutr J. 2004; 3: 9

22. Larsen, T M et al. 'Diets with high or low protein content and glycemic index for weight-loss maintenance', N Engl J Med 2010; 363(22): 2102–13

23. Halton, T L et al. 'The Effects of High Protein Diets on Thermogenesis, Satiety and Weight Loss: A Critical Review', J Am CollNutr 2004; 23(5): 373–85

24. Vinknes, K J et al. 'Dietary Intake of Protein Is Positively Associated with Percent Body Fat in Middle-Aged and Older Adults', J. Nutr 2011; 141(3): 440–46

25. O'Dea, K. 'Marked improvement in carbohydrate and lipid metabolism in diabetic Australian aborigines after temporary reversion to traditional lifestyle', Diabetes 1984; 33(6): 596–603

26. O'Dea, K. 'Westernisation, insulin resistance and diabetes in Australian aborigines', Med J Aust 1991; 155(4): 258–64

27. Daniel, M et al. 'Diabetes incidence in an Australian aboriginal population: an 8-year follow-up study', Diabetes Care 1999; 22: 1993–98

28. Lindeberg, S et al. 'Cardiovascular risk factors in a Melanesian population apparently free from stroke and ischaemic heart disease: the Kitava study', J Intern Med 1994; 236: 331–40

29. Gannon, M C, Nuttall, F Q. 'Control of blood glucose in type 2 diabetes without weight loss by modification of diet composition', *Nutrition & Metabolism* 2006; 3: 16

30. Avena, N M. 'Examining the addictive-like properties of binge eating using an animal model of sugar dependence', *ExpClinPsychopharmacol* 2007; 15(5): 481–91

31. Dallman, M F. 'Stress-induced obesity and the emotional nervous system', *Trends EndocrinolMetab* 2010; 21(3): 159–65

32. Felig, P. 'Insulin is the mediator of feeding–related thermogenesis: insulin resistance and/or deficiency results in a thermogenic defect which contributes to the pathogenesis of obesity', *Clin Physiol* 1984; 4(4): 267–73

33. Lindgärde, F. 'Traditional versus agricultural lifestyle among Shuar women of the Ecuadorian Amazon: effects on leptin levels', *Metabolism* 2004; 53(10): 1355–58

34. Simopoulos, A P. 'The Mediterranean Diets: What Is So Special about the Diet of Greece? The Scientific Evidence', *J. Nutr* 2001; 131: 3065S–3073S

35. Hite, A H. 'Low-Carbohydrate Diet Review: Shifting the Paradigm', *NutrClinPract* June 2011; 26(3): 300–308

36. Kristen, G et al. 'Lifestyle Factors and 5-Year Abdominal Fat Accumulation in a Minority Cohort: The IRAS Family Study', *Obesity* 2011; 171

37. Freed, D L J. 'Do dietary lectins cause disease? The evidence is suggestive – and raises interesting possibilities for treatment', *BMJ* 1999; 318(7190): 1023–24

38. Jönsson, T et al. 'Agrarian diet and diseases of affluence – Do evolutionary novel dietary lectins cause leptin resistance?', *BMC Endocrine Disorders* 2005; 5: 10

39. Ruales, J. 'Saponins, phytic acid, tannins and protease inhibitors in quinoa (Chenopodium quinoa, Willd) seeds', *Food Chemistry* 1993; 48(2) 137–43

40. Macfarlane, B J et al. 'Inhibitory effect of nuts on iron absorption', *Am J ClinNutr* 1988 Feb; 47(2): 270–74

41. Tuntawiroon, M. 'Rice and iron absorption in man', *Eur J ClinNutr* 1990; 44(7): 489–97

42. Kelsay, J L. 'A review of research on effects of fiber intake on man', *Am J ClinNutr* 1978; 31(1): 142–59

43. Reddy, N R et al. *Food Phytates* (CRC Press, 2001)

44. Reinhold, J G et al. 'Decreased Absorption of Calcium, Magnesium, Zinc and Phosphorus by Humans due to Increased Fiber and Phosphorus Consumption as Wheat Bread', *J. Nutr* 1976; 106(4): 493–503

45. Famularo, G et al. 'Probiotic lactobacilli: an innovative tool to correct the malabsorption syndrome of vegetarians?', *Med Hypotheses* 2005; 65(6): 1132–35

46. van Dam, R M et al. 'Dietary patterns and risk for type 2 diabetes mellitus in U.S. men', *Ann Intern Med* 2002; 136(3): 201–209

47. Hemalatha, S et al. 'Influence of germination and fermentation on bioaccessibility of zinc and iron from food grains', *Eur J ClinNutr* 2007; 61(3): 342–48

48. Gautam, S et al. 'Higher bioaccessibility of iron and zinc from food grains in the presence of garlic and onion', *J Agric Food Chem* 2010; 58(14): 8426–29

49. Sartorelli, D S et al. 'High intake of fruits and vegetables predicts weight loss in Brazilian overweight adults', *Nutr Res* 2008; 28(4): 233–38

50. German, J B, Dillard, C J. 'Saturated fats: what dietary intake?', *Am J ClinNutr* 2004; 80(3): 550–59

51. Howard, B V et al. 'Low-fat dietary pattern and risk of cardiovascular disease: the Women's Health Initiative Randomized Controlled Dietary Modification Trial', *JAMA* 2006; 295(6): 655–66

52. Micha, R, Mozaffarian, D. 'Saturated fat and cardiometabolic risk factors, coronary heart disease, stroke, and diabetes: a fresh look at the evidence', *Lipids* 2010; 45(10): 893–905

53. Ramsden, C E et al. 'Dietary fat quality and coronary heart disease prevention: a unified theory based on evolutionary, historical, global, and modern perspectives', *Curr Treat Options Cardiovasc Med* 2009; 11(4): 289–301

54. Mozaffarian, D et al. 'Effects on coronary heart disease of increasing polyunsaturated fat in place of saturated fat: a systematic review and meta-analysis of randomized controlled trials', *PLoS Med* 2010; 23; 7(3): e1000252

55. Cordain, L. 'Saturated fat consumption in ancestral human diets: implications for contemporary intakes.' *Phytochemicals, Nutrient-Gene Interactions* (CRC Press, 2006): 115–26

56. Cordain, L et al. 'Fatty acid analysis of wild ruminant tissues: evolutionary implications for reducing diet-related chronic disease', *Eur J ClinNutr* 2002; 56(3): 181–91

57. Carrera-Bastos, P et al. 'The western diet and lifestyle and diseases of civilization', *Res Rep ClinCardiol* 2011; 2: 215–35

58. Li, Z et al. 'Dietary Factors Alter Hepatic Innate Immune System in Mice with Non-Alcoholic Fatty Liver Disease', *Hepatology* 2005

59. Cordain, L et al. 'Plant-animal subsistence ratios and macronutrient energy estimations in worldwide hunter-gatherer diets', *Am J ClinNutr* 2000; 71(3): 682–92

60. Cordain, L et al. 'The paradoxical nature of hunter-gatherer diets: meat-based, yet non-atherogenic', *Eur J ClinNutr* 2002; 56(1): S42–52

61. Micallef, M et al. 'Plasma n-3 Polyunsaturated Fatty Acids are negatively associated with obesity', *Br J Nutr* 2009; 102(9): 1370–74

62. McCombie, G et al. 'Omega-3 oil intake during weight loss in obese women results in remodelling of plasma triglyceride and fatty acids', *Metabolomics* 2009; 5(3): 363–74

63. Parra, D et al. 'A diet rich in long chain omega-3 fatty acids modulates satiety in overweight and obese volunteers during weight loss', *Appetite* 2008; 51(3): 676–80

64. Piscitelli, F et al. 'Effect of dietary krill oil supplementation on the endocannabinoidome of metabolically relevant tissues from high-fat-fed mice', *NutrMetab* 2011; 8(1): 51

65. Kuipers, R S et al. 'Estimated macronutrient and fatty acid intakes from an East African Paleolithic diet', *Br J Nutr* 2010; 104(11): 1666–87

66. Siri-Tarino, P W et al. 'Meta-analysis of prospective cohort studies evaluating the association of saturated fat with cardiovascular disease', *Am J ClinNutr* 2010; 91(3): 535–46

67. Papamandjaris, A A et al. 'Medium chain fatty acid metabolism and energy expenditure: obesity treatment implications', *Life Sci* 1998; 62(14): 1203–15

68. Mañé, J et al. 'Partial replacement of dietary (n-6) fatty acids with medium-chain triglycerides decreases the incidence of spontaneous colitis in interleukin-10-deficient mice', *J Nutr* 2009; 139(3): 603–10

69. Huang, C B et al. 'Short- and medium-chain fatty acids exhibit antimicrobial activity for oral microorganisms', *Arch Oral Biol* 2011; 56(7): 650–54

70. Thormar, H et al. 'Stable concentrated emulsions of the 1-monoglyceride of capric acid (monocaprin) with microbicidal activities against the food-borne bacteria Campylobacter jejuni, Salmonella spp., and Escherichia coli', *Appl Environ Microbiol* 2006; 72(1): 522–26

71. Batovska, D I et al. 'Antibacterial study of the medium chain fatty acids and their

1-monoglycerides: individual effects and synergistic relationships', *Pol J Microbiol* 2009; 58(1): 43–47

72. Hauenschild, A *et al*. 'Successful treatment of severe hypertriglyceridemia with a formula diet rich in omega-3 fatty acids and medium-chain triglycerides', *Ann NutrMetab* 2010; 56(3): 170–75

73. Nagao, K, Yanagita, T. 'Medium-chain fatty acids: functional lipids for the prevention and treatment of the metabolic syndrome', *Pharmacol Res* 2010; 61(3): 208–12

74. St-Onge, M P *et al*. 'Medium chain triglyceride oil consumption as part of a weight loss diet does not lead to an adverse metabolic profile when compared to olive oil', *J Am CollNutr* 2008; 27(5): 547–52

75. Hite, A H *et al*. 'In the face of contradictory evidence: Report of the Dietary Guidelines for Americans Committee', *Nutrition* 2010; 26(10): 915–24

76. Hsu, Y C, Ip, M M. 'Conjugated linoleic acid-induced apoptosis in mouse mammary tumor cells is mediated by both G protein coupled receptor-dependent activation of the AMP-activated protein kinase pathway and by oxidative stress', *Cell Signal* 2011 [Epub ahead of print]

77. Kanaya, N, Chen, S. 'Conjugated linoleic acid reduces body weight gain in ovariectomized female C57BL/6J mice', *Nutr Res* 2010; 30(10): 714–21

78. Joseph, S V *et al*. 'Trans-8, cis-10+ cis-9, trans-11-conjugated linoleic acid mixture alters body composition in Syrian golden hamsters fed a hypercholesterolaemic diet', *Br J Nutr* 2010; 104(10): 1443–49

79. Dervishi, E *et al*. 'The forage type (grazing vs hay pasture) fed to ewes and the lamb gender affect fatty acid profile and lipogenic gene expression in LM of suckling lambs', *J Anim Sci* 2011 [Epub ahead of print]

80. Pribila, B A *et al*. 'Improved lactose digestion and intolerance among African-American adolescent girls fed a dairy-rich diet', *J Am Diet Assoc* 2000; 100(5): 524–28

81. Tuula, *et al*. 'Lactose Intolerance', *Journal of the American College of Nutrition* 2000; 19: 165S–175S

82. Itan, Y *et al*. 'The Origins of Lactase Persistence in Europe', *PLoS Computational Biology* 2009; 5(8): e1000491

83. Hoppe, C *et al*. 'High intakes of milk, but not meat, increase s–insulin and insulin resistance in 8-year-old boys', *Eur J ClinNutr* 200; 59(3): 393–98

84. Bulhões, A C *et al*. 'Correlation between lactose absorption and the C/T−13910 and G/A−22018 mutations of the lactase-phlorizin hydrolase (LCT) gene in adult-type hypolactasia', *Brazilian Journal of Medical and Biological Research* 2007; 40(11): 1441–46

85. Simopoulos, A P. 'The Mediterranean Diets: What Is So Special about the Diet of Greece? The Scientific Evidence', *J. Nutr* 2001; 131: 3065S–3073S

86. Anderson, D C. 'Assessment and nutraceutical management of stress-induced adrenal dysfunction', *Integrative Medicine* 2008; 7(5): 18–25

87. Aschoff, J *et al*. 'Meal timing in humans during isolation without time cues', *J Biol Rhythms* 1986; 1(2): 151–62

88. Cugini, P *et al*. 'Chronobiometric identification of disorders of hunger sensation in essential obesity: therapeutic effects of dexfenfluramine', *Metabolism* 1995; 44(2): 50–56

89. Smolensky, M, Lamberg, L. *The Body Clock Guide to Better Health* (Holt, 2000)

90. Weingarten, H P *et al*. 'Food cravings in a college population', *Appetite* 1991; 17: 167–75

91.   Rada, P et al. 'Daily bingeing on sugar repeatedly releases dopamine in the accumbens shell', *Neuroscience* 2005; 134(3): 737–44

Chapter 4 – 6 Weeks to De-Stress Success

1.   Uematsu, T et al. 'Effect of dietary fat content on oral bioavailability of menatetrenone in humans', *J Pharm Sci* 1996; 85(9): 1012–16

2.   Shin, J S et al. 'Indole-Containing Fractions of Brassica rapa Inhibit Inducible Nitric Oxide Synthase and Pro-Inflammatory Cytokine Expression by Inactivating Nuclear Factor-Kb', *J Med Food* 2011 [Epub ahead of print]

3.   Karen-Ng, L P et al. 'Combined Effects of Isothiocyanate Intake, Glutathione s-Transferase Polymorphisms and Risk Habits for Age of Oral Squamous Cell Carcinoma Development', *Asian Pac J Cancer Prev* 2011; 12(5): 1161–66

4.   Hursel, R, Westerterp-Plantenga MS. 'Thermogenic ingredients and body weight regulation', *Int J Obes* 2010; 34(4): 659–69

5.   Diepvens, K et al. 'Obesity and thermogenesis related to the consumption of caffeine, ephedrine, capsaicin, and green tea', *Am J PhysiolRegulIntegr Comp Physiol* 2007; 292(1): R77–85

6.   Pal, S, Lim, S. 'The effect of a low glycaemic index breakfast on blood glucose, insulin, lipid profiles, blood pressure, body weight, body composition and satiety in obese and overweight individuals: a pilot study', *J Am CollNutr* 2008; 27(3): 387–93

7.   Setting the scientific record straight on humanity's evolutionary prehistoric diet and ape diets. Part 2 of our Visit with Ward Nicholson. http://www.beyondveg.com accessed August 2011

8.   Bocarsly, M E et al. 'Rats that binge eat fat-rich food do not show somatic signs or anxiety associated with opiate-like withdrawal: Implications for nutrient-specific food addiction behaviors', *PhysiolBehav* 2011 [Epub ahead of print]

9.   Bulhões, A C et al. 'Correlation between lactose absorption and the C/T–13910 and G/A–22018 mutations of the lactase-phlorizin hydrolase (LCT) gene in adult-type hypolactasia', *Braz J Med Biol Res* 2007; 40(11): 1441–46

10.   deVrese, M et al. 'Probiotics–compensation for lactase insufficiency', *Am. J. Clin Nutr* 2001; 73 (2): 421S–429S

11.   Simopoulos, A P. 'The Mediterranean Diets: What Is So Special about the Diet of Greece? The Scientific Evidence', *J. Nutr* 2001; 131: 3065S–3073S

12.   Braun, L, Cohen, M. *Herbs & Natural Supplements. An evidence-based guide* (2nd edn; Churchill, 2007)

13.   Anderson, D C. 'Assessment and nutraceutical management of stress-induced adrenal dysfunction', *Integrative Medicine* 2008; 7(5): 18–25

14.   Cordain, L. 'The nutritional characteristics of a contemporary diet based upon Paleolithic food groups', *J Am Nutraceut Assoc* 2002; 5: 15–24

15.   Li, Y et al. 'Effects of multivitamin and mineral supplementation on adiposity, energy expenditure and lipid profiles in obese Chinese women', *Int J Obes* 2010; 34(6): 1070–77

16.   Major, G C et al. 'Multivitamin and dietary supplements, body weight and appetite: results from a cross-sectional and a randomised double-blind placebo-controlled study', *Br J Nutr* 2008; 99(5): 1157–67

17. Kimmons, J E et al. 'Multivitamin use in relation to self–reported body mass index and weight loss attempts', *MedGenMed* 2006; 8(3): 3

18. Pizzorno, J E, Murray, M T. *Textbook of Natural Medicine* (3rd edn; Churchill Livingstone, 2010)

19. Office of Dietary Supplements. *Dietary Supplement Fact Sheet: Vitamin C* (Health Professional). US National Institutes of Health http: //ods.od.nih.gov/factsheets/ VitaminC-HealthProfessional accessed August 2011

20. Micallef, M et al. 'Plasma n–3 Polyunsaturated Fatty Acids are negatively associated with obesity', *Br J Nutr* 2009; 102(9): 1370–74

21. Werbach, M R. 'Nutritional Strategies for Treating Chronic Fatigue Syndrome', *Alternative Medicine Review* 2000; 5(2): 93–108

22. Sawazaki, S et al. 'The effect of docosahexaenoic acid on plasma catecholamine concentrations and glucose tolerance during longlasting psychological stress: a double-blind placebo-controlled study', *J NutrSciVitaminol* 1999; 45(5): 655–65

23. Hamazaki, T et al. 'The effect of docosahexaenoic acid on aggression in young adults. A placebo-controlled double-blind study', *J Clin Invest* 1996; 97: 1129–33

24. Delarue, J et al. 'Fish oil prevents the adrenal activation elicited by mental stress in healthy men', *Diabetes Metab* 2003; 29(3): 289–95

25. Piscitelli, F et al. 'Effect of dietary krill oil supplementation on the endocannabinoidome of metabolically relevant tissues from high-fat-fed mice', *NutrMetab* 2011; 8(1): 51

26. Kiecolt-Glaser, J K. 'Omega-3 supplementation lowers inflammation and anxiety in medical students: A randomized controlled trial', *Brain, Behavior, and Immunity* 2011 [Epub ahead of print]

27. Kidd, P M. 'Omega-3 DHA and EPA for cognition, behavior, and mood: clinical findings and structural-functional synergies with cell membrane phospholipids', *Altern Med Rev* 2007; 12(3): 207–27

28. Famularo, G et al. 'Probiotic lactobacilli: an innovative tool to correct the malabsorption syndrome of vegetarians?', *Med Hypotheses* 2005; 65(6): 1132–35

29. Ley, R E et al. 'Microbial ecology: Human gut microbes associated with obesity', *Nature* 2006; 444:1022–23

30. Kadooka, Y et al. 'Regulation of abdominal adiposity by probiotics (Lactobacillus gasseri SBT2055) in adults with obese tendencies in a randomized controlled trial', *Eur J ClinNutr* 2010; 64(6): 636–43

31. Messaoudi, M et al. 'Assessment of psychotropic-like properties of a probiotic formulation (Lactobacillus helveticus R0052 and Bifidobacteriumlongum R0175) in rats and human subjects', *British Journal of Nutrition* 2011; 105: 755–64

32. Ka, S O et al. 'Silibinin attenuates adipogenesis in 3T3–L1 preadipocytes through a potential upregulation of the insig pathway', *Int J Mol Med* 2009; 23(5): 633–37

33. Anderson, D C. 'Assessment and nutraceutical management of stress-induced adrenal dysfunction', *Integrative Medicine* 2008; 7(5): 18–25

34. Morgan, M, Bone, K. 'Herbs to enhance energy and performance, a phytotherapist's perspective', *Mediherb* 2008; 124

35. Rada, P et al. 'Daily bingeing on sugar repeatedly releases dopamine in the accumbens shell', *Neuroscience* 2005; 134(3): 737–44

36. Hoebel, B G et al. 'Evidence for sugar addiction: Behavioral and neurochemical effects of intermittent, excessive sugar intake', *Neuroscience and Biobehavioral Reviews* 2008; 32: 20–39

37. Erlanson-Albertsson, C. 'Sugar triggers our reward-system. Sweets release opiates which stimulates the appetite for sucrose – insulin can depress it', *Lakartidningen* 2005; 102(21): 1620–22

38. Blass, E *et al.* 'Interactions between sucrose, pain and isolation distress', *PharmacolBiochem Behav* 1987; 26(3): 483–89

39. Warne, J P. 'Shaping the stress response: interplay of palatable food choices, glucocorticoids, insulin and abdominal obesity', *Mol Cell Endocrinol* 2009; 300(1–2): 137–46

40. Wideman, C H *et al.* 'Implications of an animal model of sugar addiction, withdrawal and relapse for human health', *NutrNeurosci* 2005 ; 8(5–6): 269–76

41. Wintola, O A *et al.* 'The effect of Aloe ferox Mill. in the treatment of loperamide-induced constipation in Wistar rats', *BMC Gastroenterol* 2010; 10: 95

42. Jönsson, T *et al.* 'Paleolithic diet is more satiating per calorie than a Mediterranean-like diet in individuals with ischemic heart disease', *NutrMetab* 2010; 7(1): 85

43. Manzano, S, Williamson, G. 'Polyphenols and phenolic acids from strawberry and apple decrease glucose uptake and transport by human intestinal Caco-2 cells', *Molecular Nutrition & Food Research* 2010; 54(12): 1773–80

44. Torronen, R *et al.* 'Berries modify the postprandial plasma glucose response to sucrose in healthy subjects', *Br J Nutr* 2010; 103(8): 1094–97

45. Amo, K *et al.* 'Effects of xylitol on metabolic parameters and visceral fat accumulation', *J ClinBiochemNutr* 2011; 49(1): 1–7

46. Jarvill-Taylor, K J *et al.* 'A hydroxychalcone derived from cinnamon functions as a mimetic for insulin in 3T3–L1 adipocytes', *J Am CollNutr* 2001 Aug; 20(4): 327–36

47. DesMaisons, K. *Potatoes Not Prozac* (Simon & Schuster, 2008)

48. Tylka, T L. 'Development and psychometric evaluation of a measure of intuitive eating', *Journal of Counseling Psychology* 2006; 53(2): 226–40

49. Hairston, K G *et al.* 'Lifestyle Factors and 5-Year Abdominal Fat Accumulation in a Minority Cohort: The IRAS Family Study', *Obesity* 2011 [Epub ahead of print]

50. Hemalatha, S *et al.* 'Influence of germination and fermentation on bioaccessibility of zinc and iron from food grains', *Eur J ClinNutr* 2007; 61(3): 342–48

51. Di Cagno, R *et al.* 'Proteolysis by sourdough lactic acid bacteria: effects on wheat flour protein fractions and gliadin peptides involved in human cereal intolerance', *Appl Environ Microbiol* 2002; 68: 623–33

52. Avena, N M, Hoebel, B G. 'A diet promoting sugar dependency causes behavioral cross-sensitization to a low dose of amphetamine', *Neuroscience* 2003; 122(1): 17–20

Chapter 5 – A Breakfast Revolution

1. Timlin, M T. 'Breakfast Eating and Weight Change in a 5-Year Prospective Analysis of Adolescents: Project EAT (Eating Among Teens)', *Pediatrics* 2008; 3: e638–e645

2. Rampersaud, G C *et al.* 'Breakfast habits, nutritional status, body weight, and academic performance in children and adolescents', *J Am Diet Assoc* 2005; 105(5): 743–60

3. Blom, W A M *et al.* 'Effect of a high-protein breakfast on the postprandial ghrelin response', *Am J ClinNutr* 2006; 83(2): 211–20

4. Kapur, S *et al.* 'Postprandial Insulin and Triglycerides after Different Breakfast Meal Challenges: Use of Finger Stick Capillary Dried Blood Spots to Study Postprandial Dysmetabolism', *J Diabetes SciTechnol* 2010; 4(2): 236–43

5. Tin, S P et al. 'Breakfast skipping and change in body mass index in young children', Int J Obes 2011; 35(7): 899–906
6. Vander Wal, J S et al. 'Egg breakfast enhances weight loss', Int J Obes 2008; 32(10): 1545–51
7. Ratliff, J et al. 'Consuming eggs for breakfast influences plasma glucose and ghrelin, while reducing energy intake during the next 24 hours in adult men', Nutr Res 2010; 30(2): 96–103
8. Dhurandhar, N V et al. 'Egg breakfast enhances weight loss', FASEB J 2007; 21: 538
9. Isaksson, H et al. 'Effect of rye bread breakfasts on subjective hunger and satiety: a randomized controlled trial', Nutr J 2009 Aug 26; 8: 39
10. Neustadt, J. 'Mitochondrial Dysfunction and Disease', Integrative Medicine 2006; 5(3): 14–20
11. Molyneux, S M et al. 'Coenzyme Q10: Is There a Clinical Role and a Case for Measurement?', Research Review 2008; 29(2): 71–82
12. Mizuno, K et al. 'Antifatigue effects of coenzyme Q10 during physical fatigue', Nutrition 2008; 24(4): 293–99

Chapter 6 – The Building Blocks of Lunch and Dinner

1. Duckett, S K. 'Understanding Factors Affecting Meat Quality – Results from Pasture Based Beef Systems – 3 year multi State Study', American Grassfed Association, 2007
2. Freedman, N D et al. 'Association of meat and fat intake with liver disease and hepatocellular carcinoma in the NIH–AARP cohort', J Natl Cancer Inst 2010; 102(17): 1354–65
3. Micha, R et al. 'Red and processed meat consumption and risk of incident coronary heart disease, stroke, and diabetes mellitus: a systematic review and meta-analysis', Circulation 2010; 121(21): 2271–83
4. Williams, D E et al. 'Xenobiotics and xenoestrogens in fish: modulation of cytochrome P450 and carcinogenesis', Mutation Research/Fundamental and Molecular Mechanisms of Mutagenesis 1998; 399(2): 179–92
5. Popular Seafood: Best & Worst Choices. Environmental Defense Fund. 2011 http://apps.edf.org/page.cfm?tagID=1521 accessed August 2011
6. List of Seafood Health Alerts. Environmental Defense Fund. 2011 http://apps.edf.org/page.cfm?tagID=17694 accessed August 2011
7. Kastel, M A. 'Maintaining the Integrity of Organic Milk', The Cornucopia Institute. Presented to the USDA National Organic Standards Board, 2006
8. Butler, G et al. 'Fat composition of organic and conventional retail milk in northeast England', J Dairy Sci 2011; 94(1): 24–36
9. Puotinen, C J. 'Unhealthy Vegetable Oils? Does Food Industry Ignore Science Regarding Polyunsaturated Oils? Implications for Cancer, Heart Disease', Well Being Journal 2005; 14(3)
10. Block, E. 'The Chemistry of Garlic and Onion', Sci Am 1985; 252: 94–99
11. Gautam, S et al. 'Influence of combinations of promoter and inhibitor on the bioaccessibility of iron and zinc from food grains', Int J Food SciNutr 2011 [Epub ahead of print]

12. Gautam, S et al. 'Higher bioaccessibility of iron and zinc from food grains in the presence of garlic and onion', *J Agric Food Chem* 2010; 58(14): 8426–29

13. Layrisse, M et al. 'New property of vitamin A and B carotene on human iron absorption: effect on phytate and polyphenols as inhibitors of iron absorption', *ArchivosLatinoamericanos de Nutricion* 2000; 50(3)

14. Chrispeels, M J, Raikel, N V. 'Lectins, lectin genes, and their role in plant defense', *Plant Cell* 1991; 3: 1–9

15. Hemalatha, S et al. 'Influence of germination and fermentation on bioaccessibility of zinc and iron from food grains', *Eur J ClinNutr* 2007; 61(3): 342–48

16. Gautam, S et al. 'Influence of combinations of promoter and inhibitor on the bioaccessibility of iron and zinc from food grains', *Int J Food SciNutr* 2011 [Epub ahead of print]

17. Hemalatha, S et al. 'Influence of heat processing on the bioaccessibility of zinc and iron from cereals and pulses consumed in India', *J Trace Elem Med Biol* 2007; 21(1): 1–7

18. Nachbar, M S et al. 'Lectins in the United States diet: a survey of lectins in commonly consumed foods and a review of the literature', *Am J Clin Nutr* 1980; 33(11): 2338–45

Chapter 7 – Taking the Stress Out of Lunch

1. Research carried out in 2009 by Spar

2. Research carried out by Warburtons July 2009

3. Johnson, C S. 'Strategies for Healthy Weight Loss: From Vitamin C to the Glycaemic Response', *Journal of the American College of Nutrition* 2005; 24(3): 158–65

Chapter 8 – De-Stressing Dinner

1. Head, K, Kelly, G. 'Nutrients and botanicals for treatment of stress: Adrenal fatigue, neurotransmitter imbalance, anxiety, and restless sleep', *Alt. Med. Rev* 2009; 14(2): 114–40

2. Backhaus, J et al. 'Sleep disturbances are correlated with decreased morning awakening salivary cortisol', *Psychoneuroendocrinology* 2004; 29 (9): 184–91

3. Cutolo, M et al. 'Circadian rhythms: Glucocorticoids and arthritis', *Ann. NY Acad. Sci* 2006; 1069: 289–99

4. Yang, X. 'A wheel of time: the circadian clock, nuclear receptors, andphysiology', *Genes Dev* 2010; 24: 741–47

5. Smolensky, M, Lamberg, L. *The Body Clock Guide to Better Health* (Holt, 2000)

6. Shang, Y et al. 'Imaging analysis of clock neurons reveals light buffers the wake-promoting effect of dopamine', *Nat Neurosci* 2011; 14(7): 889–95

7. Mollicone, D J et al. 'Optimizing sleep/wake schedules in space: Sleep during chronic nocturnal sleep restriction with and without diurnal naps', *ActaAstronautica* 2007; 60(4–7): 354–61

8. Office of Dietary Supplements. *Dietary Supplement Fact Sheet: Magnesium* (Health Professional). US National Institutes of Health http://ods.od.nih.gov/factsheets/Magnesium–HealthProfessional accessed August 2011

9. Murck, H. 'Magnesium and affective disorders', *NutrNeurosci* 2002; 5(6): 375–89

10. Cernak, I et al. 'Alterations in magnesium and oxidative status during chronic emotional stress', *Magnes-Res* 2000; 13(1): 29–36

11. Seelig, M S. 'Consequences of magnesium deficiency on the enhancement of stress reactions; preventive and therapeutic 68 implications (a review)', *Journal of the American College of Nutrition* 1994; 13(5): 429–46

12. Galan, P et al. 'Dietary magnesium intake in a French adult population', *Magnesium Research* 1997; 10(4): 321–28

13. Quaranta, S et al. 'Pilot study of the efficacy and safety of a modified-release magnesium 250 mg tablet (Sincromag) for the treatment of premenstrual syndrome', *Clin Drug Investig* 2007; 27(1): 51–58

14. Sole, M J et al. 'Diurnal physiology: core principles with application to the pathogenesis, diagnosis, prevention, and treatment of myocardial hypertrophy and failure', *Journal of Applied Physiology* 2009; 107(4): 1318–27

15. Winkelman, J W. 'Reduced Brain GABA in Primary Insomnia: Preliminary Data from 4T Proton Magnetic Resonance Spectroscopy (1H–MRS)', *Sleep* 2008; 31(11): 1499–1506

16. Abdou, A M et al. 'Relaxation and immunity enhancement effects of gamma-aminobutyric acid (GABA) administration in humans', *Biofactors* 2006; 26(3): 201–208

17. Yoo, D Y et al. 'Pyridoxine enhances cell proliferation and neuroblast differentiation by upregulating the GABAergic system in the mouse dentate gyrus', *Neurochem Res* 2011; 36(5): 713–21

18. Bromek, E et al. 'Cytochrome P450 mediates dopamine formation in the brain in vivo', *J Neurochem* 2011; 118(5): 806–15

19. Smolensky, M, Lamberg, L. *The Body Clock Guide to Better Health* (Holt, 2000)

20. Beck, M E. 'Dinner Preparation in the United States', *British Food Journal* 2007; 109(7): 531–47

21. Holt, S H A et al., 'A Satiety Index of Common Foods', *European Journal of Clinical Nutrition* 1995: 675–90

22. Braun, L, Cohen, M. *Herbs & Natural Supplements. An evidence-based guide* (2nd edn; Churchill, 2007)

23. Ko, F N et al. 'Vasodilatory action mechanisms of apigenin isolated from Apiumgraveolens in rat thoracic aorta', *BiochimBiophysActa* 199; 1115(1): 69–74

Chapter 9 – Stress-free Drinks and Snacks

1. Duffey, K J, Popkin, B M. 'Energy Density, Portion Size, and Eating Occasions: Contributions to Increased Energy Intake in the United States, 1977–2006', *PLoS Med* 2011; 8(6): e1001050

2. Blom, W A M et al. 'Effect of a high-protein breakfast on the postprandial ghrelin response', *Am J ClinNutr* 2006; 83(2): 211–20

3. Ifland, J R et al. 'Refined food addiction: a classic substance use disorder', *Med Hypotheses* 2009; 72(5): 518–26

4. Ledochowski, M et al. 'Fructose malabsorption is associated with decreased plasma tryptophan', *Scand. J. Gastroenterol* 2001; 36 (4): 367–71

5. UT Southwestern Medical Center. 'Limiting Fructose May Boost Weight Loss, Researcher Reports', *ScienceDaily*, 2008

6. Fernandes et al. 'Mouse study: Aspartame consumption in diabetes-prone mice', The University of Texas Health Science Center San Antonio 2011 http://www.uthscsa.edu/hscnews/singleformat2.asp?newID=3861 accessed August 2011

7. Yang, Q. 'Gain weight by "going diet?" Artificial sweeteners and the neurobiology of sugar cravings', Yale J Biol Med 2010; 83(2): 101–108

8. http://education.wichita.edu/caduceus/examples/soda/tbspn_in_can.html accessed August 2011

9. Hazuda, H P. 'Human study: The San Antonio Longitudinal Study of Aging', The University of Texas Health Science Center San Antonio 2011 http://www.uthscsa.edu/hscnews/singleformat2.asp?newID=3861 accessed August 2011

10. Francesco, S et al. 'Taste perception and implicit attitude toward sweet related to body mass index and soft drink supplementation', Appetite 2011; 57: 237–46

11. http://www.ipsos-mori.com/researchpublications/researcharchive/1982/Chocolate-Pushes-Sex-Into-Second-Place.aspx accessed August 2011

12. Buitrago-Lopez, A et al. 'Chocolate consumption and cardiometabolic disorders: systematic review and meta-analysis', BMJ 2011; 343: d4488

13. Drewnowski, A et al. 'Taste responses and preferences for sweet high-fat foods: evidence for opioid involvement', PhysiolBehav 1992; 51(2): 371–79

14. Martin, F P et al. 'Metabolic Effects of Dark Chocolate Consumption on Energy, Gut Microbiota, and Stress-Related Metabolism in Free-Living Subjects', J. Proteome Res 2009; 8(12): 5568–79

15. Tey, S L et al. 'Nuts improve diet quality compared to other energy-dense snacks while maintaining body weight', J NutrMetab 2011: 357350

16. Cassady, B A et al. 'Mastication of almonds: effects of lipid bioaccessibility, appetite and hormone response', Am J. Clin Nut 2009; 89: 794–800

17. McCartney. 'Waterlogged?', BMJ 2011; 343: d4280.

18. Saat, M et al. 'Rehydration after exercise with fresh young coconut water, carbohydrate-electrolyte beverage and plain water', J PhysiolAnthropolAppl Human Sci 2002; 21(2): 93–104

19. O'Keefe, J H, Cordain, L. 'Cardiovascular Disease Resulting From a Diet and Lifestyle at Odds With Our Paleolithic Genome: How to Become a 21st-century Hunter-Gatherer', Mayo Clin Proc 2004; 79: 101–10

20. Anderson, D C. 'Assessment and nutraceutical management of stress-induced adrenal dysfunction', Integrative Medicine 2008; 7(5): 18–25

21. Powers, S K, Dodd, S. 'Caffeine and endurance performance', Sports Med 1985; 2(3): 165–74

22. Armstrong, L E. 'Caffeine, Body Fluid–Electrolyte Balance, and Exercise Performance', International Journal of Sport Nutrition & Exercise Metabolism 2002; 12: 189–206

23. Smillie, L D, Gökçen, E. 'Caffeine enhances working memory for extraverts', Biol Psychol 2010 Dec; 85(3): 496–98

24. Amin, N et al. 'Genome-wide association analysis of coffee drinking suggests association with CYP1A1/CYP1A2 and NRCAM', Mol Psychiatry 2011 Aug 30. [Epub ahead of print]

25. Al-Qarawi, A et al. 'Liquorice (Glycyrrhizaglabra) and the adrenal–kidney–pituitary axis in rats', Food Chem2002; 40(10): 1525–27

26. Hammer, F, Stewart, P M. 'Cortisol metabolism in hypertension', Best Pract Res ClinEndocrinolMetab 2006; 20(3): 337–53

27. Soon-Jae, R. 'Green tea catechin improves microsomal phospholipase A$_2$ activity and the arachidonic acid cascade system in the kidney of diabetic rat', *Asia Pacific J ClinNutr* 2002; 11(3): 226–31

28. Park, K S et al. '(−)–Epigallocatethin–3–O–gallate counteracts caffeine-induced hyperactivity: evidence of dopaminergic blockade', *BehavPharmacol* 2010 Sep; 21(5–6): 572–75

29. Higashiyama, A et al. 'Effects of l–theanine on attention and reaction time response', *Journal of Functional Foods* 2011; 3(3): 171–78

30. Survey of caffeine levels in hot beverage April 2004 http://www.food.gov.uk/multimedia/pdfs/fsis5304.pdf accessed August 2011

31. Kim, S et al. 'Resveratrol exerts anti-obesity effects via mechanisms involving down-regulation of adipogenic and inflammatory processes in mice', *BiochemPharmacol* 2011; 81(11): 1343–51

32. Simopoulos, A P. 'The Mediterranean Diets: What Is So Special about the Diet of Greece? The Scientific Evidence', *J. Nutr* 2001; 131: 3065S–3073S

33. Cargiulo, T. 'Understanding the health impact of alcohol dependence', *American Journal of Health-System Pharmacy* 2007 ; 64(5,3): S5–S11

34. Oscar-Berman, M, Marinkovic, K. 'Alcoholic Brain Damage', *Alcohol Research & Health.* 2003; 27(2): 125–33

35. Spreckelmeyer, K N. 'Opiate-Induced Dopamine Release Is Modulated by Severity of Alcohol Dependence: An [(18)F]Fallypride Positron Emission Tomography Study', *Biol Psychiatry* 2011 Jul. [Epub ahead of print]

36. Mishra, D, Chergui, K. 'Ethanol inhibits excitatory neurotransmission in the nucleus accumbens of adolescent mice through GABA(A) and GABA(B) receptors', *Addict Biol* 2011 Jul. [Epub ahead of print]

Chapter 10 – The New Mind–Body Movement

1. Hassmen, P et al. 'Physical Exercise and psychological well-being: a population study in Finland', *Preventative Medicine* 2000; 30(1): 17–25

2. Harvard Women's Health Watch, December 2006

3. Cox, R et al. 'Effects of Acute Bouts of Aerobic Exercise of Varied Intensity on Subjective Mood Experiences of Women of Different Age Groups Over Time', *Journal of Sport Behaviour* 2006

4. Cordain, L et al. 'Physical Activity, Energy Expenditure and Fitness: An Evolutionary Perspective', *International Journal of Sports Medicine* 1998; 19(5): 328–35

5. Biddle, S et al. *Physical Activity and Psychological Wellbeing* (Routledge, 2000)

6. Lydon, C. *Ten Years Thinner* (Mobius, 2008)

7. Boutcher, S H. 'High Intensity Intermittent Exercise and Fat Loss', *J Obes* 2011: 865305

8. Trapp, E G et al. 'The effects of high intensity intermittent exercise training on fat loss and fasting insulin levels of young women', *International Journal of Obesity* 2008; 32(4): 684–91

9. Jakicic, J M et al. 'Effect of exercise on 24 month weight loss maintenance in overweight women', *Archives of Internal Medicine* 2008; 168(14): 1550–59

10. Tremblay, M S et al. 'Incidental movement, lifestyle-embedded activity and sleep: new frontiers in physical activity assessment', *Can J Public Health* 2007; 98(2): S208–17

References

11. Tudor-Locke, C et al. 'How many steps/day are enough?', *Sports Medicine* 2004; 34(1): 1–8

12. Kusher, R F et al. 'The PPET Study: People and Pets Exercising Together', *Obesity* 2006; 14(10): 1762–70

13. Boreham, C A G et al. 'Training effects of short bouts of stair climbing on cardiorespiratory fitness, blood lipids, and homocysteine in sedentary young women', *British Journal of Sports Medicine* 2005; 39(9): 590–93

14. Boyd, S, Eaton, M B. *The Paleolithic Prescription: A Program of Diet & Exercise and a Design for Living* (Harper Collins, 1989)

15. O'Keefe, J et al. 'Achieving Hunter-gatherer Fitness in the 21st Century: Back to the Future', *Amer J Med* 2010; 123(12): 1082–86

16. Wilson, M et al. 'Diverse patterns of myocardial fibrosis in lifelong, veteran endurance athletes', *J Appl Physiol* 2011; 110(6): 1622–26

17. Edlund, M. *The Power of Rest: Why Sleep Alone Is Not Enough. A 30-Day Plan to Reset Your Body* (HarperOne, 2011). Quoted with kind permission from the author

18. Bach, B et al. 'A comparison of muscular tightness in runners and non-runners and the relation of muscular tightness to low back pain in runners', *Journal of Orthopedic Sports Physical Therapy* 1985; 6: 315–23

19. Corbin, C B et al. 'Flexibility: A major component of physical fitness', *The Journal of Physical Education and Recreation* 1980; 51: 23–24, 57–60

20. DeVries, H A et al. 'EMG comparison of single doses of exercise and meprobamate as to effects of muscular relaxation', *American Journal of Physical Medicine* 1972; 51: 130–41

21. DeVries, H A et al. 'Tranquilizer effect of exercise', *American Journal of Physical Medicine* 1981; 60: 57–66

22. Jeffrey, R et al. 'A Time Series Diary Study of Mood and Social Interaction', *Motivation and Emotion* 1998; 22

23. Hull, E et al. 'Effects of dance on physical and psychological wellbeing in older persons', *Archives of Gerontology and Geriatrics* 2009; 49(1): e45–50

24. Hall, S A et al. 'Sexual activity, erectile dysfunction and incident cardiovascular events', *American Journal of Cardiology* 2010; 105(2): 192–97

25. Ebrahim, S et al. 'Sexual intercourse and risk or ischaemic stroke and coronary heart disease: the Caerphilly study', *Journal of Epidemiological Community Health* 2002; 56(2): 99–102

26. Goldenberg, M et al. 'Why Individuals Hike the Appalachian Trail: A Qualitative Approach to Benefits', *Journal of Experiential Education*. 2008; 30(3): 277–81

27. Hideo, N et al. 'Effect of negative air ions on computer operation, anxiety and salivary chromogranin A-like immunoreactivity', *IntJournPsychophys* 2002; 46: 85–89

28. Ramagopalan, S V et al. 'A ChIP-seq defined genome-wide map of vitamin D receptor binding: Associations with disease and evolution', *Genome Research* 2010; 20

29. Holick, M F. 'The Vitamin D Epidemic and its Health Consequences', *J Nutr* 2005; 135: 2739S–2748S

30. Pretty, J et al. 'A Countryside for Health and Well-Being: The Physical and Mental Health Benefits of Green Exercise', Report for the Countryside Recreation Network, February 2005.

31. Teas, J et al. 'Walking Outside Improves Mood for Healthy Postmenopausal Women', *Oncology* 2007; 1: 35–43

32. Sami, L et al. 'Drop-out and mood improvement: a randomised controlled trial with light exposure and physical exercise', *BMC Psychiatry* 2004; 4: 22
33. Wouter, D et al. 'Cold-Activated Brown Adipose Tissue in Healthy Men', *N Engl J Med* 2009; 360: 1500–1508

Chapter 11 – Calm for Life

1. Kristal, A R. 'Yoga practice is associated with attenuated weight gain in healthy, middle-aged men and women', *AlternTher Health Med* 2005; 11(4): 28–33
2. Farhi, D. *The Breathing Book: Vitality and Good Health Through Essential Breath Work* (Holt, 1996)
3. Conti, P B. 'Assessment of the body posture of mouth–breathing children and adolescents', *J Pediatr (Rio J)* 2011; 87(4): 357–63
4. Conrad, A. 'Psychophysiological effects of breathing instructions for stress management', *ApplPsychophysiol Biofeedback* 2007; 32(2): 89–98
5. Gallup, A C, Gallup, G G Jr. 'Yawning and thermoregulation', *PhysiolBehav* 2008; 95(1–2): 10–16
6. Vlemincx, E. 'Sigh rate and respiratory variability during mental load and sustained attention', *Psychophysiology* 2011; 48(1): 117–20
7. Matta, C. 'Can Meditation Lower Your Risk for Heart Disease?' http://blogs.psychcentral.com/dbt/2011/07/can–meditation–lower–your–risk–for–heart–disease/ accessed August 2011
8. Davidson, R J, Lut, A. 'Buddha's Brain: Neuroplasticity and Meditation'. *IEEE Signal Processing Magazine* 2007; 172–76
9. Kaul, P. 'Meditation acutely improves psychomotor vigilance, and may decrease sleep need', *Behavioral and Brain Functions* 2010; 6: 47
10. Sivasankaran, S. 'The Effect of a Six-Week Program of Yoga and Meditation on Brachial Artery Reactivity: Do Psychosocial Interventions Affect Vascular Tone?', *Clin. Cardiol* 2006; 29,: 393–98
11. Kamei, T et al. 'Decrease in serum cortisol during yoga exercise is correlated with alpha wave activation', *Percept Mot Skills* 2000; 90(3,1): 1027–32
12. Wheeler, A, Wilkin L. 'A Study of the Impact of Yoga Âsana on Perceived Stress, Heart Rate, and Breathing Rate', *International Journal of Yoga Therapy* 2007; 17: 57–63
13. Telles, S et al. 'Short term health impact of a yoga and diet change program on obesity', *Med SciMonit* 2010; 16(1): CR35–40
14. Field, T. 'Yoga clinical research review', *Complementary Therapies in Clinical Practice* 2010: 1–8
15. Wheeler, A. 'The Impact of Bi-weekly Yoga Classes on Menstrual Cycle of College-Aged Females', Department of Kinesiology, California State University CA. Submitted for publication http://onesourceyoga.com/page8/page20/page20.html
16. Wheeler, A. 'The Effects of T. Krishnamacharya Style Yoga Class on Body Image of Female College Students', Department of Kinesiology, California State University CA. Submitted for publication http://onesourceyoga.com/page8/page19/page19.html accessed August 2011
17. Field, T. 'Yoga clinical research review', *Complementary Therapies in Clinical Practice* 2010: 1–8

18. Wheeler, A. 'An Analysis of Personality, Yoga Preferences and the Relaxation Response', paper presented at the International Association of Yoga Therapy Sytar Conference, 2007, Los Angeles, CA

19. Carei, T R. 'Randomized controlled clinical trial of yoga in the treatment of eating disorders', *J Adolesc Health* 2010; 46(4): 346–51

20. McIver, S. '"Overeating is not about the food": women describe their experience of a yoga treatment program for binge eating', *Qual Health Res.* 2009; 19(9): 1234–45

21. Streeter, C C. 'Yoga Asana Sessions Increase Brain GABA Levels: A Pilot Study', *J Altern Complement Med* 2007; 13(4): 419–26

22. Kiecolt-Glaser, J. 'Stress, Inflammation, and Yoga Practice', *Psychosomatic Medicin* 2010; 72(2): 113–21

BIBLIOGRAPHY

Baer, R A. *Mindfulness-Based Treatment Approaches: A clinician's guide to evidence base and applications* (Academic Press, 2005)

Biddle, S et al. *Physical Activity and Psychological Wellbeing* (Routledge, 2000)

Boyd, S, Eaton, M B. *The Paleolithic Prescription: A Program of Diet & Exercise and a Design for Living* (Harper Collins, 1989)

DesMaisons, K. *Potatoes Not Prozac* (Simon & Schuster, 2008)

Edlund, M. *The Power of Rest: Why sleep alone is not enough* (HarperCollins, 2010)

Farhi, D. *The Breathing Book: Vitality and Good Health Through Essential Breath Work* (Holt, 1996)

Glenville, M. *Mastering Cortisol: Stop Your Body's Stress Hormone from Making You Fat Around the Middle* (Amorata Press, 2006)

Hanh, T.N. *The Miracle of Mindfulness: The Classic Guide to Meditation by the World's Most Revered Master* (Rider, 2008)

Kaminoff, L. *Yoga Anatomy: Your illustrated guide to postures, movements, and breathing techniques* (Human Kinetics Europe Ltd, 2007)

Kessler, D. *The End of Overeating: Taking control of our insatiable appetite* (Penguin, 2010)

Long, R. *Scientific Keys Volume I: The Key Muscles of Hatha Yoga* (3rd edn; Bandha Yoga, 2006)

McClellan, S, Hamilton, B. *So Stressed* (Simon & Schuster, 2010)

Pizzorno J E, Murray M T. *Textbook of Natural Medicine* (3rd edn; Churchill Livingstone, 2010)

Sapolsky, R M, *Why Zebras Don't Get Ulcers* (Holt, 2004)

Smolensky, M, Lamberg, L. *The Body Clock Guide to Better Health* (Holt, 2000)

Stiles, M. *Structural Yoga Therapy: Adapting to the Individual* (Red Wheel/Weiser, 2000)

Wansink, J. *Mindless Eating* (Hay House, 2011)

Weatherby, D. *Signs and Symptoms Analysis from a Functional Perspective* (2nd edn; Weatherby & Associates, LLC, 2004)

Wilson, J. *Adrenal Fatigue, the 21st Century Stress Syndrome* (Smart Publications, 2002)

INDEX

The index is in word-by-word order which takes account of spaces, so 'exercise technique' comes before 'exercises'.

Enjoyed *The De-Stress Diet?*

Register today for the free De-Stress Diet email and podcast support programme during your 6-Week Plan

For extra nutrition, exercise and wellbeing advice, log on to:

de-stressyourlife.com

You will find:

- real-time videos of De-Stress Diet yoga sequences and strength workouts that can be downloaded onto your iPad, mp3 player, Smartphone or laptop

- recommended food suggestions and easy ordering to make your De-Stress Diet journey easier

- information on trusted suppliers and nationwide resources for all your De-Stress Diet needs

- up-to-date research, interviews and discussion from leading nutrition, fitness and De-Stress experts

PLUS

Sign up for the De-Stress Your Life monthly newsletter and receive a FREE Expert Support tool

ABOUT THE AUTHORS

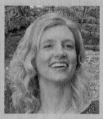 **Charlotte Watts** is a nutritional therapist with over ten years' experience. She trained at The Institute for Optimum Nutrition in London, where she was later a tutor and year programme leader. She now lectures at the College of Naturopathic Medicine UK. As well as a private practice, Charlotte also consults for corporate clients and health companies, giving talks and workshops. She has been the nutritionist/presenter on BBC3's *Freaky Eaters* and on GMTV. She writes for national magazines, is often quoted in the press and has written and consulted on many nutritional books. Charlotte is also a 500-hour Yoga Alliance trained teacher with the Vajrasati School of Yoga, Brighton, and combines this skill for a holistic approach to health issues. She has been teaching yoga classes, workshops and corporate events and writing on the subject for over four years, with a 15-year practice. She lives in Brighton with her partner, Sam, and their daughter, Maisie. More info at charlottewattshealth.com

Fitness consultant **Charlene Hutsebaut** is a certified personal trainer with 20 years experience in the fitness industry, holding degrees in both Physical Education and Education. She is certified with the National Strength and Conditioning Association, holds a REPs Level 3 certificate (UK) and is a Stott-certified pilates instructor.

Nutritional cooking consultant **Tina Deubert** is a nutritional therapist, Bowen therapist and keen cook. She has run a farmers' market and is the author of *The Friendly Vegetable Book*, designed to give families ideas for using more locally produced, seasonal vegetables.

ABOUT THE AUTHORS

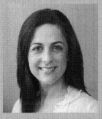

Anna Magee is a multi-award winning health journalist whose clients include *Australian Good Health* and *Body & Soul* (*Sunday Telegraph*) Magazine along with UK *Marie Claire*, the *Daily Mail*, *The Sun*, *Woman & Home* and *Grazia*.

Currently based in the UK, Anna is Contributing Editor on *Red magazine* and Health Editor on Sainsbury's Magazine, the UK's leading supermarket supplement. Anna writes a blog called Thinking Women's Health at annamagee.wordpress.com and she has three awards for journalism, the most recent of which was for Best Consumer Magazine Feature in the Guild of Health Writers Awards for a piece in UK *Marie Claire*.

Born and bred in Australia, Anna began her career on newspapers in Sydney before moving to monthly magazines. She holds a Bachelor's degree in English from the University of Sydney and a post-graduate diploma in journalism from the University of Technology.

Anna moved to the UK in 2003 and spent four-and-a-half years as Health Director on *Red magazine*. She now remains contributing editor on Red and is also Health Editor on Sainsbury's magazine. Anna also produces online video content specialising in health and lifestyle.

Prior to living in the UK, Anna lived in Ireland for four and a half years where she was health correspondent for *Image* magazine and health writer for the *Irish Independent's Weekend Magazine* as well as *FeelGood*, the health supplement with the *Irish Examiner*.

Anna now lives in East London with her partner Kevin Magee, a TV producer and cameraman. *The De-Stress Diet* is her first book. Anna also does limited editorial and corporate consulting on a contract basis. Find out more about Anna's journalism and view her portfolio at www.annamagee.com

We hope you enjoyed this Hay House book. If you'd like to receive our online catalogue featuring additional information on Hay House books and products, or if you'd like to find out more about the Hay Foundation, please contact:

Hay House Australia Pty. Ltd.,
18/36 Ralph St., Alexandria NSW 2015
Phone: 612-9669-4299 *Fax:* 612-9669-4144
www.hayhouse.com.au

Published and distributed in the United States by:
Hay House, Inc., P.O. Box 5100, Carlsbad, CA 92018-5100
(760) 431-7695 or (800) 654-5126
(760) 431-6948 (fax) or (800) 650-5115 (fax)
www.hayhouse.com® • **www.hayfoundation.org**

Published and distributed in the United Kingdom by: Hay House UK,
Ltd., 292B Kensal Rd., London W10 5BE • *Phone:* 44-20-8962-1230
Fax: 44-20-8962-1239 • www.hayhouse.co.uk

Published and distributed in the Republic of South Africa by:
Hay House SA (Pty), Ltd., P.O. Box 990, Witkoppen 2068
Phone/Fax: 27-11-467-8904 • www.hayhouse.co.za

Published in India by: Hay House Publishers India, Muskaan Complex,
Plot No. 3, B-2, Vasant Kunj, New Delhi 110 070 • *Phone:* 91-11-4176-
1620 • *Fax:* 91-11-4176-1630 • www.hayhouse.co.in

Distributed in Canada by: Raincoast, 9050 Shaughnessy St.,
Vancouver, B.C. V6P 6E5 • *Phone:* (604) 323-7100
Fax: (604) 323-2600 • www.raincoast.com

Take Your Soul on a Vacation

Visit **www.HealYourLife.com®** to regroup, recharge, and reconnect
with your own magnificence. Featuring blogs, mind-body-spirit news,
and life-changing wisdom from Louise Hay and friends.

Visit **www.HealYourLife.com** today!